"For the people in Porto of Prince Haiti there is a God above we must put our trust and faith in him"

HOPE FOR HAITI

CHEF B.D WILLIAMS OFFICIAL SALAD BOOK LIKE YOU'VE NEVER SEEN BEFORE

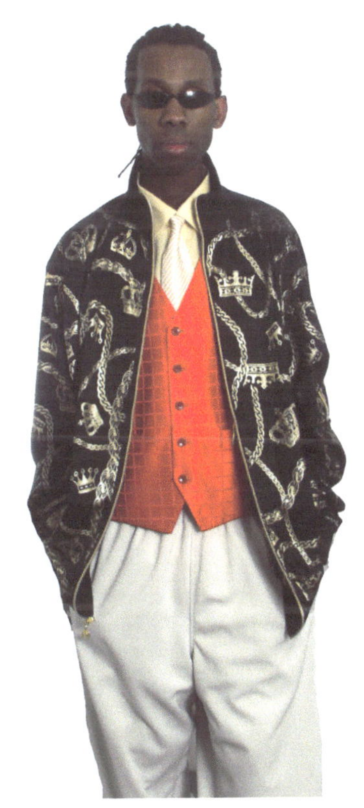

A Chef of Great Reputation

BRIAN DAVID WILLIAMS

Order this book online at www.trafford.com
or email orders@trafford.com

Most Trafford titles are also available at major online book retailers.

Information: www.chefubsenterprise.com & www.housedreamshopefoundation.com
Send your comments to www.Facebook.ca/ Chef B.D Williams
Printed in the United States of America.

ISBN: 978-1-4269-3555-8

Library of Congress Control Number: 2010909380

Trafford rev. 06/09/2011

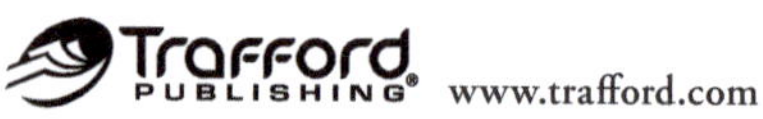

www.trafford.com

North America & international
toll-free: 1 888 232 4444 (USA & Canada)
phone: 250 383 6864 • fax: 812 355 4082

Together we can make a difference; it's never too late to reach out and helped those in need, we must come together like one.

~ THIS BOOK IS USED FOR RAISING FUNDS TO

HELP THE PEOPLE OF HAITI THANK YOU...

Contents

PREFACE

For most of my life while working as an apprentice learning how to cook throughout the restaurants here in Montreal Canada, I must say; I have came a long way to achieving a great deal of knowledge. I have gone through many rocky roads that sometimes it had accord to me that I was never going to be successful in it. It is a gift from God that I have became somebody able to understand what I needed to do, for me to be able to inspired others in what started out as a dream to me, now here I am working successfully in what makes me happy, and yet nothing could ever come closed to my feeling of creating dishes of lovely salads. It's a joy that comes from my heart for me to learn such a wonderful art, and now I have decided to used what I learn to help others in need in a time of crisis. The pictures of salads that are including in my book, including the recipes were done as I was working on making salads. I did not invent these recipes, what I have done is added my own taste and my own unique style with creativeness. And while I was practicing at home I gain other ideas for making my own signature salads, which will be use for only my business as I will be opening soon. I have been risking my whole life all these years so that I can create my own part in this world, this is my part and I thank all my teachers who helped me get there. I am Chef Brian David Williams, whose autobiography will soon be available as well.

"My love for cooking comes from the inside, with love and creativeness, and today;
I am reaching out for the people of Haiti with what I know how to do best."
Chef BD. Williams.

The people's Chef B.D. WILLIAMS autobiography is soon to be available, the behind story of a man willing to do what it takes to achieve success.

Chefubsenterprise.com catalog of salad and ingredients book is created by chef B D Williams, the people's chef, while putting together this book and getting ready for publication, the news of a terrible earthquake had aroused in Haiti, and had struck me surprisingly, deaths unfolded, homes were lost, kids were left helpless and in pain.

I then turned my attention towards helping the people of Haiti, my way of contributing, helping to raise funds, let's give hope and love to the people of Haiti, all sales from this book well be donated to CanadaHopeforHaiti.ca.

www.chefubsenterprise.com is a cooking site of great reputation, the founder of this cooking site is chef B.D Williams who is currently working on creating a Charitable Foundation (House Dreams Hopes Where Dreams Begin). You can be sure of finding pictures of salads on chefubsenterprise.com. For more information on the author and how you can purchase his books, you can search for him on the worldwide web.

I usually prepared everything I did in advance making salads easier to make during busy working schedule.

Chef B.D WILLIAMS GREEK Potato Salad

First boil potatoes (half tender not completely cooked)

Then cut potatoes into cubes place olive oil

2 tbsp of oreganos herbs

1 tbsp of salt and black pepper

Chopped fresh parsley include

Sprinkle a dash of paprika powder

Place in oven to completely bake

Cut red or yellow sweet peppers and green sweet peppers

Cut shallots and include leave to garnish

Tried Chef B.D Williams delightful work of Salads (B.D Williams specialties)

The best of Chef B.D Williams and his love for creating Salads recipes shows in his works.

Always prepared a dish while memorizing the recipe in your mind

Chef B.D Williams Masala Potato Salad

Take natural potatoes slice or dice and seasoning with salt and black pepper ¼ cup of vegetable oil or olive oil

Bake in Oven 350 degrees 15 too 20 minutes until you get a golden color

Take another frying pan and sauté vegetables, long yellow beans and green beans baby carrots including other spices, a dash of black sesame seed, a tsp of salt and black pepper. A tsp of chili flakes Add a tsp of turmeric while sautéing. A tsp of grind Masala that comes in a pack, you can purchase Shan Masala in Indian stores or supermarkets.

Finely chopped parsley and mix inside the potatoes

Be sure to mix all the spices and potatoes together and serve ready either hot or cold.

Masala is usually a mixed of spices such as, cardamom, bark, cloves, cumin, black pepper, nutmeg and cinnamon, a little dash of turmeric and of course food coloring.

I tried to give others the best in making salads as I came too learned so gratefully. These salads are very simple to make with an eye catching feeling. You be amazed what you can get out of simplicities. And yes I am thankful for learning such an art it is an honor.

CHEF B.D WILLIAMS BEETS SALAD

First boil Beets (Do not boiled beets too soft but tender enough to be eatable) Then peeled Beets and cut into cubes or half moon

Add ½ cup of sugar depending on the amount of beets
Add ¼ cup of balsamic vinegar
Add ¼ cup of red wine Vinegar
Add dash of black pepper and salt
Add 1 tbsp or 2 tbsp of lemon juice or real lime juice is better
Add fresh chopped parsley and top it off with oranges peeled and cut into half-moon.

Use pieces of oranges and parsley for garnishing.

CHEF B.D WILLIAMS RICE SALAD

Cook the rice to be eatable, (not too hard and not too soft)

Add in the rice 2 tbsp of oil, a dash of cumin seeds and turmeric curry powder for taste and colored

Five to six tomatoes dice thinly
2 too 3 onions finely chopped
Chopped a handful of fresh parsley
Sauté onions in oil for 5 minutes
Add dice tomatoes in sauté onions
Add one pack of Masala in what is sautéing

Stirred all together and let them cooked for 10 to 15 minutes

Add 1 cup of fresh dice chicken and allowed it to simmer

Poor what is sauté into cooked rice and mixed all together

Garnish with slice tomatoes half moon, parsley, chives or shallots including yellow or red peppers.

CHEF B. D WILLIAMS SPINACH SALAD

One or two fresh fennel cut julienne
One Fresh whole purple cabbage cut julienne
One fresh whole Chinese white cabbage cut julienne
Two or three whole red peppers cut julienne
2 handful of mixed lettuce leaves
2 handful of baby spinach
A dash of black pepper
1 tsp of salt
½ cup of sugar
½ cup of balsamic vinegar
½ cup of vegetable oil
2 tbsp of red wine vinegar

Mixed ½ cup of sugar, balsamic vinegar and vegetable oil in a bowl, be sure to stir using a wisp until liquid is puree. And the dash of black pepper red wine vinegar and mixed. Place the sauce in the bowl of vegetables and mixed together.

First of all this is how I figured out how to make Pesto Pasta Salad
1st take a stainless steel pot add as much water to cover the Pasta

I usually add 2 small bowl of pasta to make a full bowl and a half

Add Pasta once the water is boiling, do not over cooked the Pasta, it will loose the shape.

Once the Pasta is ready set aside and allowed it to simmer or wash it in cold water.

Take a bowl or deep cup and puree all these ingredients, use a kitchen aid electrical blender please for better consistency.

Add 2 tbsp of salt
Add 1 tbsp of black pepper
Add handfuls of fresh basil
Add a handful of spinach
Add handful of fresh parsley
Add a dash of dry oregano
And used olive oil to help blend these herbs

(Optional) Some people do use nuts and other choices

This is what I usually do:

Once all these are blended it becomes green and the spinach makes its even greener. Mixed this pesto sauce with the Penne and taste for a bit of salt and black pepper be sure you feel it at your throat. Now add a handful of parmesan cheese.

Then take a handful of sundried tomatoes finely slice them or dice place inside the salad and decorate with finishing touch and you are ready to serve.

CHEF B.D WILLIAMS GREEK SALAD

I was giving an advice to walk with my camera with me while working, a friend offered me this idea after seeing my passion for making salads, now this is what I called my signature salads.

Take a bowl that you prefer, this is my way of showing you what it looks unique and simple.

Take 2 or 3 bunches of Roman leaves and cut into pieces bite sizes
Take a few whole tomatoes fresh and dice them into cubes place aside for décor and it's eatable.
Take a few cucumbers and dice them into cubes and place them aside as well.

You can then portion them out by layers

Place Roman at the bottom of the bowl

Then add slices of tomatoes and cucumbers set aside

Then repeat the same dilemma, add tomatoes and cucumbers

To finish off add olives and feta

Sprinkle with oregano

Don't forget to use Greek dressing to top it off when serving others and your self.

CHEF B.D WILLIAMS LENTIL SALAD

I always create different salads that allow me to give other people something more eye catching. Some salads I offered other examples.

Boil lentil must be tender not too soft

Wash lentil in cold water and let it drain

Chopped a bunch of shallots
Cut red and green peppers into cubes
Take one whole cucumber and great it inside
One or two carrots great inside as well
Add a tbsp of black pepper and salt
Add a quarter cup of olive oil for flavoring

Mixed all ingredients together with lentil decorate a plate with lettuce leaf and slice tomatoes (optional)

Spinach Salad with Fennel after preparing in a bowl

Fresh Spinach leaves, fennel cut julienne, grated carrots, purple cabbage and Spanish cabbage cut julienne. And red peppers cut julienne always remember people eat with their eyes.

Ingredients

2 tbsp of balsamic vinegar or ¼ cup depending on how much you are making
¼ cup of red wine vinegar
¼ cup of olive oil or vegetable (optional)
¼ cup of rice wine vinegar
1½ cup of sugar
2 tsp salt and black pepper

Optional ¼ cup of natural plum sauce

Chef B.D Williams Chick Peas and Mix Beans Salad Including black Beans to top it off.

Usually you can purchased any of these mix beans at any local supermarkets

Open one cans of mix Beans precooked

One can of Chick Peas precooked

Take measuring cup measure the amount of black beans 1 ½ or 2 ½ cups placed to boiled until soft and tender add a tbsp spoon of salt for taste.

Take a bowl and add all the beans together

Add ¼ cup of lemon juice depending on the amount of beans
Add 2 tsp of salt and black pepper
Take 2 Red peppers and 2 green peppers dice it up into cubes including them into the mix beans
Add ¼ cup of vegetable oil or olive oil

Sprinkle turmeric curry non spicy curry just a little to give coloring

Orzo Salad made from Spinach and Cranberries

Boil Orzo in stainless pat make sure the water comes at a boiling temperature before adding. You can get this Orzo wheat in any local markets.

Cooked Orzo wheat only for 10 too 12 minutes while stirring it consistently to prevent from sticking.

Once it is done allowed it to strain in cold water, let the water sift through the orzo as much as possible for it to have an eatable taste.

Now you should be ready to make this salad

Add ¼ cup of olive oil into deep bowl
1 tsp of salt and black pepper
Add a handful of spinach
Add a handful of cranberries
Add a handful of capers
Add a handful of mash feta
Add fresh parsley fincly chopped
Add a handful of chicken breast already oven baked

Now mix all these ingredients with Orzo taste for salt and if possible black pepper. Garnish the top with little feta and cranberries, dice oven roasted chicken and place as well.

Vegetable Salad make with Artichoke using the other ingredients as describe.

Broccoli florets cut into finger sizes and set aside in a bowl
Cauliflower florets cut into finger sizes and set aside in a bowl
Red and green peppers also cut into cubes set aside
Carrots also cut aside and set aside

Dressing ingredients

From any can of artichoke which you can purchased in any store, strain artichoke water and set aside

Take a large mixing bowl add
¼ cup of Olive oil or vegetable
2 tbsp of white sugar (no brown sugar)
2 tsp of salt and black pepper
2 tbsp of dry or fresh oregano
¼ cup of lemon juice or just enough for taste

Now what I do to substitute, I would add ¼ cup of plum sauce dressing ¼ cup of Thai sesame dressing which you can purchased in any local grocery store. Add in bowl and mixed together. Serve cold as these are cold salads.

Vegetable Waldorf salad make with Apples

This is just a simple salad with of course all fresh veggies nothing here is cooked.

Broccoli florets cut into finger pieces and set aside in a bowl
Cauliflower florets cut into finger pieces and set aside in a bowl
Red and green peppers also cut into cubes set aside
Carrots also cut aside and set aside
Zucchini can be added or small plum tomatoes (optional)

There are times when I would either add red apples or fennel.
And there are times when I would add fresh artichokes or what I think can color it up a bit with healthy stuff, salads are nutritious food according to how you look at it.

Dressing ingredients

¼ cup of Olive oil
2 tbsp of white sugar
2 tsp of salt and black pepper
2 tbsp of dry or fresh oregano
¼ cup of lemon juice or just enough for taste
Now what I do to substitute, I would add ¼ cup of Italian dressing which you can purchased in any local grocery store.

To top it off chopped fresh parsley and mixed the vegetables in until it feels ready to eat.

Granny Smith Apples with Fennel Cranberries and Walnuts

Take Spanish purple cabbage and cut into julienne
Take granny smith apple and slice them half moon
Bake walnut in oven for 12 too 15 minutes 350 degrees while you prepare the salad in a bowl
Sometimes I do add white cabbage which stays all white looking
Add even spinach depending on what I have in the fridge

This dressing goes well with this salad

1 ½ cup of sugar or if you prefer plum sauce
¼ cup of rice wine vinegar
¼ cup of red wine vinegar
1 too tbsp of honey or in French Meil (Honey)
¼ cup of balsamic vinegar
2 tsp of salt and black pepper
Finely chopped fresh parsley

Often I use parsley for all my salads which people tense to like.
Now you can use your magic hands for mixing all these ingredients in. You want to make it a bit sour and a bit sweet. Take the walnuts and cranberries and add them inside as well as garnishing. Serve cold some salads can be serve hot depending on the person.

Chef B. D Williams Potato Salad decorated with Granny Smith Apples with grated carrots same ingredients use as in different pictures.

Chef B. D Williams Potato Salad decorated with red peppers and grated carrots same concept.

These are my favorite salads I spent endless time making them as how I imagining them to be.

These potatoes are bowled extra soft a little eatable of course, one day before and place in a cool refrigerator for better consistent.

Next day I slice them into cubes placing them in a large mixing bowl.
I then add a little olive oil, I tried using olive oil in many of my salads it may be expensive of course you can used vegetable oil.

1 tsp of salt and black pepper
2 too 3 tbsp of white sugar
2 tbsp of sour cream
¼ cup of Ranch dressing
¼ cup of coleslaw dressing
2 tbsp of regular mustard or 1 tbsp of Dijon Mustard
A dash of real lemon juice
Take 2 carrots finely grate inside as well
If you don't have carrots 2 red pepper finely dice will do the ambience as well.

Wash and prepare red apples cut them half moon and decorate in a circle around the bowl. Red apples or granny smith apples can do it as well.
Now you can mixed all these ingredients in with fresh Parsley and for garnish use the grated carrots or the dice red peppers in the middle. Serve cold and keep in the refrigerator. Have in mind cream salads do not stay along in fridges take precautions avoiding food danger.

Macaroni Salad in Red Wine Sauce

Now this is a simple ready to eat salad
I always make tomato sauce in advance using red wine. I find sauces always taste better when it is done a day in advance.

You can find tomatoes sauces recipe on www.chefubsenterprise.com and information on how you can easily make tomato sauce.
Take a stainless steel pat place on hot fire burner
Place vegetable oil inside and allowed it to get hot
Once the oil is hot add onions and sauté please do not allow the onions to get brown.
Once the onions are tender add fresh garlic, no powder garlic, (2 tbsp)
Place your dice tomatoes that come ready made in cans into the pat.

¼ cup of red wine
2 tbsp of chili flakes
Add 2 tbsp of sugar
A handful of fresh basil and parsley
A handful of dry oregano
Also you can add 1 tbsp of tomato paste (optional)
2 tsp or tbsp of salt and black pepper

Allowed the tomato sauce to cook for a 15 minutes
Use a blender and puree it.

Now this is done it's time to make the salad.

The Macaroni should be boiled in water like any Paste not too soft and not too hard. I know people love using the fancy words; but I teach you the best how I can, so you don't need to look it up in a dictionary.

Once the Macaroni is boiled and rinsed in cold water now you can add ½ cup of that tomato sauce into a bowl with the Macaroni. Now place all these other ingredients such as; dash of salt and black pepper, a handful of parmesan, fresh parsley. Take 1 or 2 small red peppers dice place inside the salad and to finish off dice sundry tomatoes. Serve as a cold salad.

Fissile Tuna Salad

You may not know this but my gift for making salads and food starts from being simple

Boil paste as I explained throughout all the salads.
Prepared a dish for mixing the salads before anything else
Take the paste and rinsed in very cold water.

Add 1¼ tbsp of vegetable oil or olive oil

Take 2 handful of tuna comes in cans and places it with the paste
Add ¼ cup of Ranch dressing
Add 2 to 4 tbsp of mayonnaise
Add 2 tsp of salt and black pepper
Chopped fresh parsley and add a handful

Corn and Mixed Bean Salad

You can purchased corns and mixed beans comes in cans in local stores
You may have to strain them and even rinsed them for a more profound taste.

Mixed the corn up with the mixed beans

Also you can purchase mixed vegetables pack comes with peas, carrots, red and green peppers other veggies is including.

On the other hand, I would dice red, green, yellow peppers and dice carrots and mixed it in with the corns and mixed beans, mostly required for my job.

Add 2 tsp salt and black pepper
Add a dash of dry oregano
Add fresh chopped parsley
¼ cup of lemon juice

Mixed all the ingredients and taste for salt and black pepper and lemon juice is required.

BONUS SALADS FROM THE CHEF

Chef B.D Williams Mushroom and Tomato Salad

A handful of ripe baby tomatoes do not sliced
1 ½ lb of fresh white mushroom sliced
Used as much green onions cut julienne
2 tbsp of capes placed whole
¼ cup of olive oil
2 too 3 tbsp of olive oil
A handful of chopped fresh coriander
A tbsp of lemon juice just for taste
2 tsp of salt and black pepper

Placed tomatoes and mushrooms in a large mixing salad bowl, now add onions and the capes; sprinkle with oil and mixed well.

Pour in the other vinaigrette and mixed again.
You can add some hard boiled eggs cut half-moon (Optional)

Chef B.D Williams tropical Fruit Salad

Take a ripe juicy Pineapple cut away the hard skin and cut into cubes bite size
Ripe papaya cut into cubes (real summer salads)
I am not a big fan of pomegranate fruit, but you can add it to your fruit bowl as well (optional)
Peel and cut some lovely juicy Florida orange into cubes

My favorite fruit watermelon cut it into bit sizes chunk

Place whole tangerines after peeling off the skin

Fresh pears, pared
2 ripe bananas cut into cubes
3 too 4 plums, pared
3 too 4 apples, pared

Fresh cantaloupe, pared

Fresh honeydew, pared

Add fresh raspberries (optional)

Fresh red and green grapes included

Mixed all the fruits together if you find not sweet enough add a bit of sugar.

Chef B.D Williams Green Family Style Salad

1 head of lettuce
1 ½ curly endive
2 tomatoes cut in wedges
3 stalk celeries cut in sticks
2 too 3 radishes, sliced (optional)
2 head of sweet onions, julienne
1 green pepper, sliced

Break lettuce head into a mixing bowl making it bite size; tear off the endive leafs and cut into small pieces. Cut tomatoes in wedges set aside for arranging on top the salad. Add celery stalks, radishes, sweet onions and green onions. My dressing was always simple,
Sprinkle a bit of balsamic vinegar, lemon juice and olive oil. Top off with tomatoes for an eye catching feeling.

Chef B.D Williams first homemade style potato salads

4 large potatoes boiled peeled and cut into cubed
1 head of green onions in French shallots finely chopped, used the white bottom part
2 tbsp of finely chopped parsley
2 tbsp of vegetable oil (until I learned olive oil was better)
1 tsp of salt and pepper
After potatoes are bowl cut into cubes
Add green onions, parsley, salt and pepper, sprinkle gently do not add too much.
Add olive oil and mixed together

This usually serve warm or cold just as good as it gets.

Chef B.D Williams Chicken Avocado Salad

½ tbsp of Tabasco sauce
¼ cup of mayonnaise
2 tbsp of real lemon juice
1 tbsp of white wine vinegar
Take ½ inch dice or slices of black forest ham,
Take a few cooked chicken breasts which are much tender; cut always into strips for greater ambiences.
3 too 4 small tomatoes, quartered
A handful of green olives sliced
2 too 3 avocados sliced
Yellow strip beans cut lengthwise

Place Tabasco sauce in bowl with the mayonnaise, add lemon juice and mix together.
Add wine vinegar and slices of black forest ham toss in chicken and mix well. Add tomatoes, green olives, and yellow strip beans including the avocados and mix well.

Take a bowl with curly lettuce and place this chicken mixture on top and now it is ready to serve. Some chicken salads such as Caesar salads recommend you place croutons; this salad goes well with avocados instead of croutons.

To learn more about chef B.D Williams and finding recipes please go to Montréal's best cooking site: www.chefubsenterprise.com

Chef B.D Williams homemade Style Maraschino Cherries Salad

2 cups of freshly drained maraschino cherries
1 cup of red or white grapes
¼ cup of cashew nuts finely crashed
½ cup of whipped cream, whipped
2 beaten egg yolks
1 tbsp of white sugar
Dash of salt (optional)

2 pared oranges, cut in pieces
2 cups of marshmallows, cut into bite sizes
3 Tablespoon of sugar

Take a large bowl, using a mixing spoon, add whipped cream, egg yolk and white sugar. Stir in sugar and mixed very well. Cut grapes and removed seeds. Add grapes, cherries, oranges marshmallows and stir well. Just before serving, place in a refrigerator and allowed to chill. Top your salad off with clusters of extra red grapes and cherries.

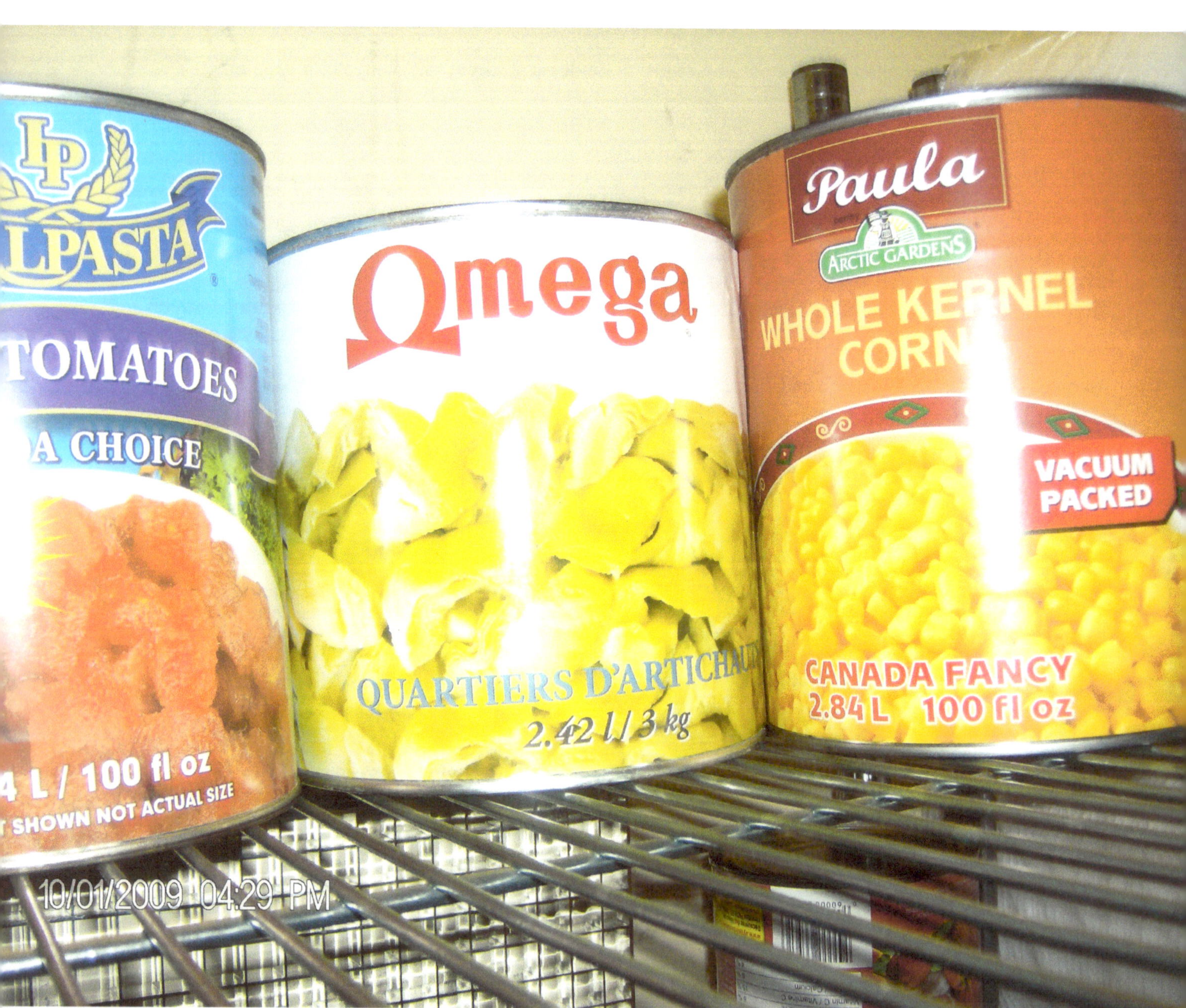
LPASTA
TOMATOES
A CHOICE
4 L / 100 fl oz
SHOWN NOT ACTUAL SIZE
Omega
QUARTIERS D'ARTICHAUTS
2.42 l / 3 kg
Paula
ARCTIC GARDENS
WHOLE KERNEL
CORN
VACUUM
PACKED
CANADA FANCY
2.84 L 100 fl oz
10/01/2009 04:29 PM

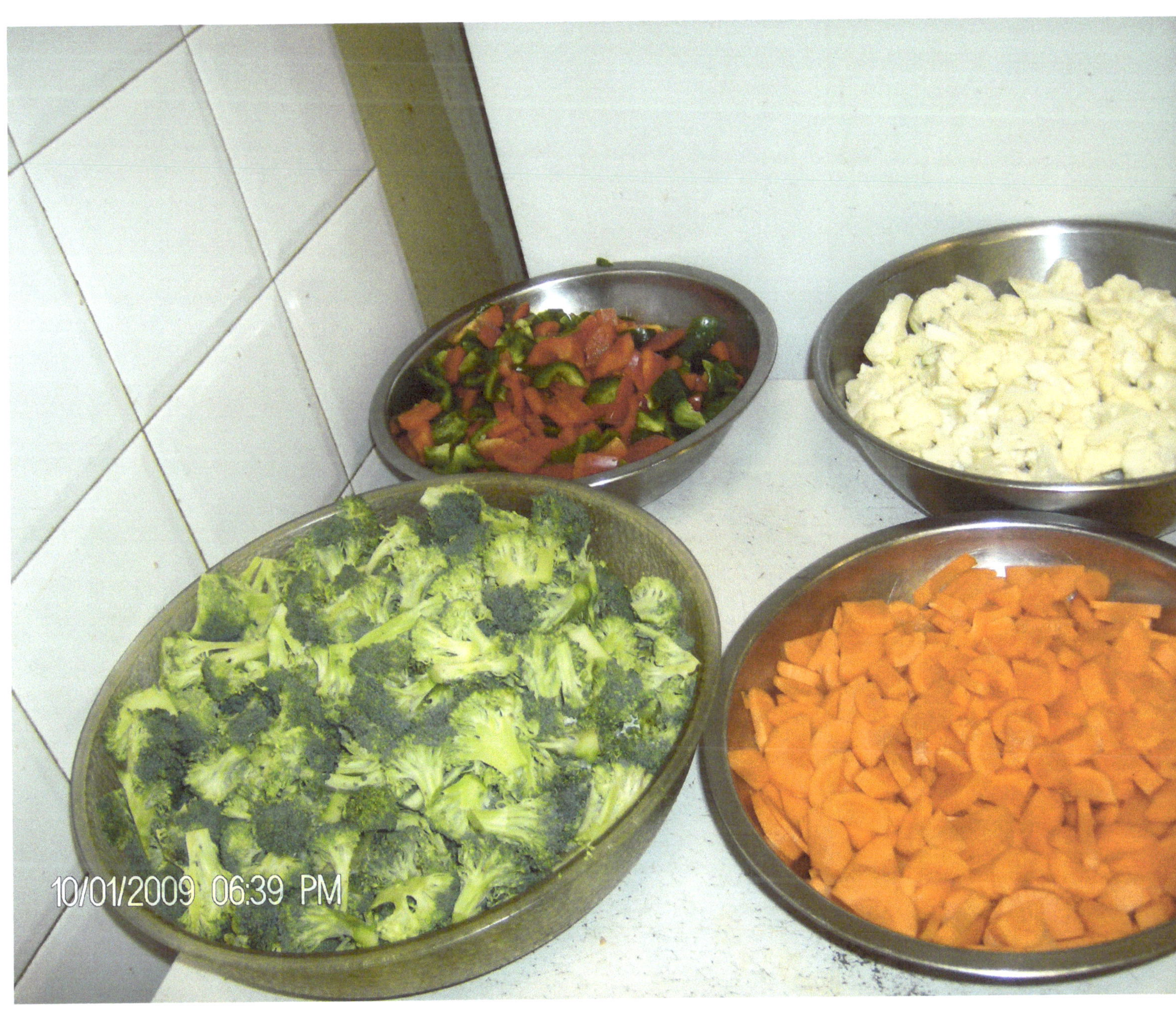
10/01/2009 06:39 PM

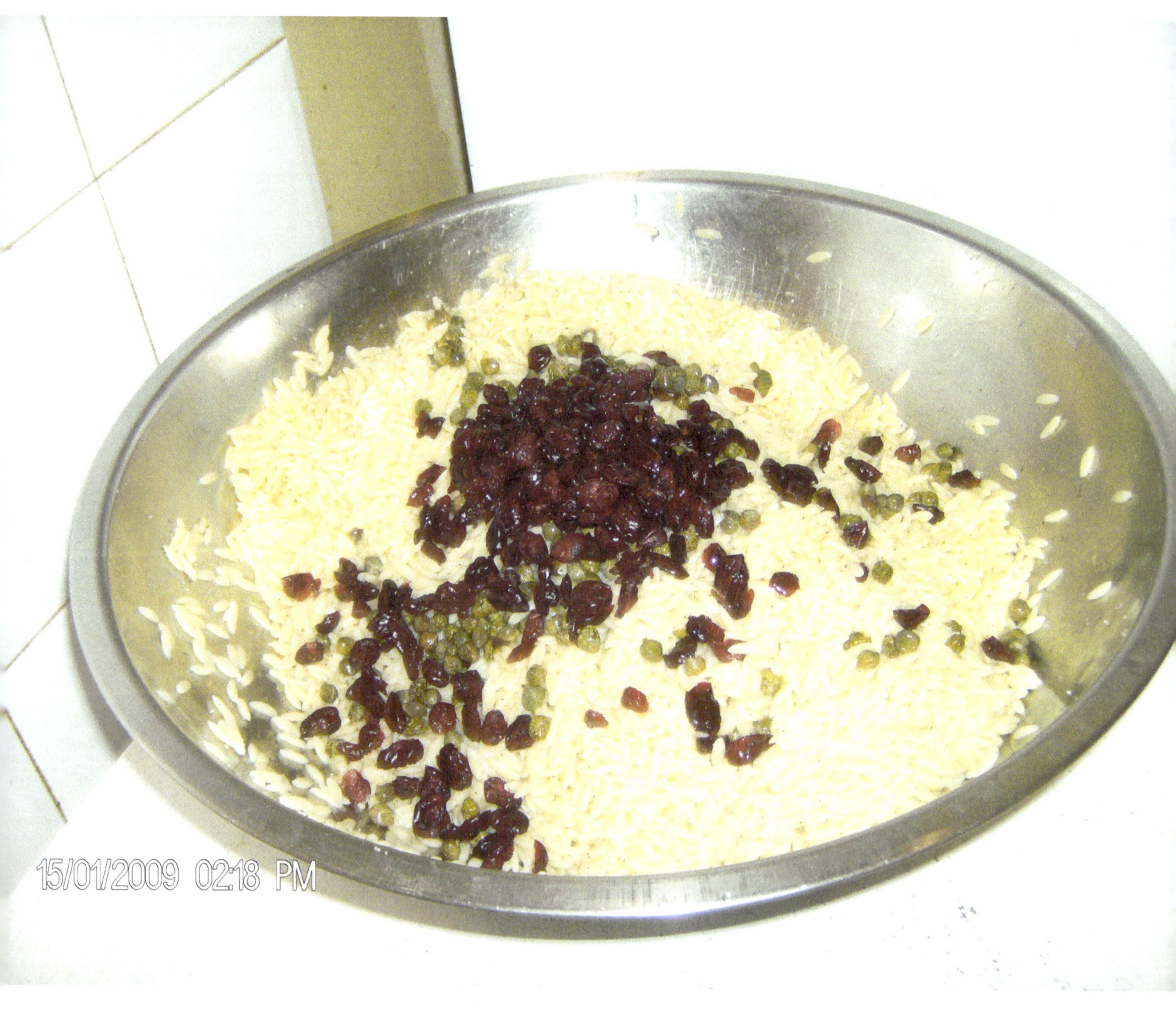
15/01/2009 02:18 PM

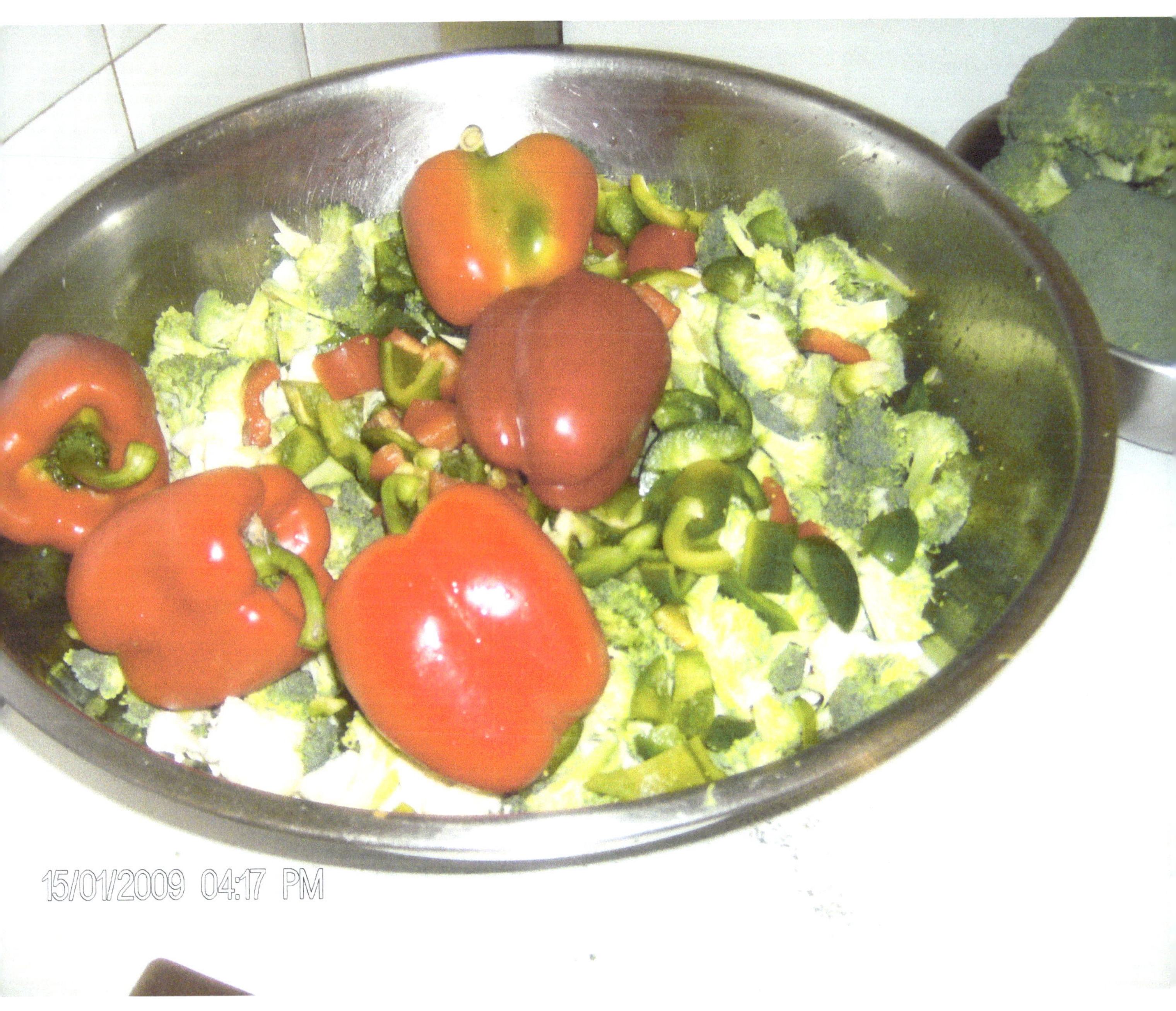
15/01/2009 04:17 PM

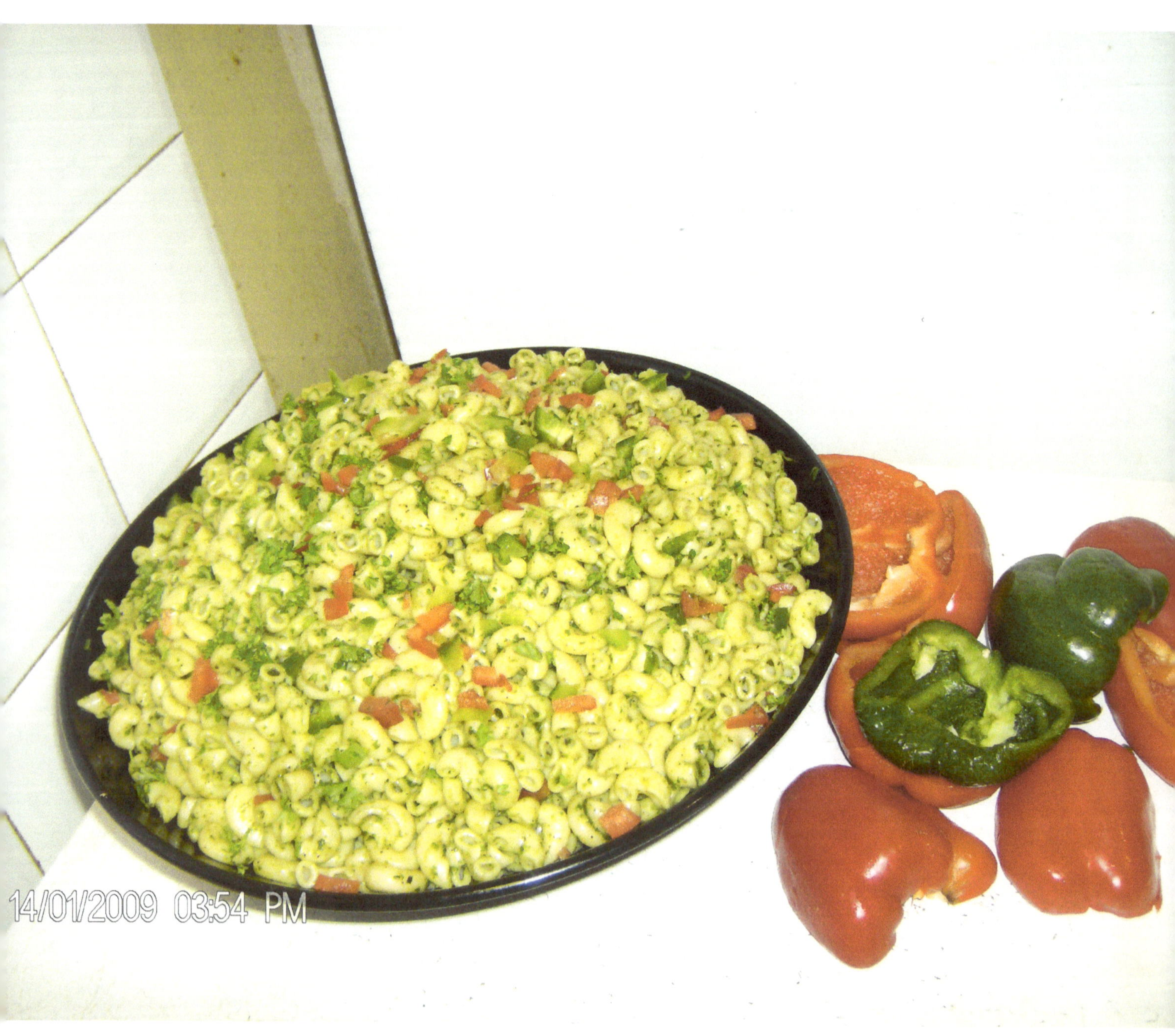
14/01/2009 03:54 PM

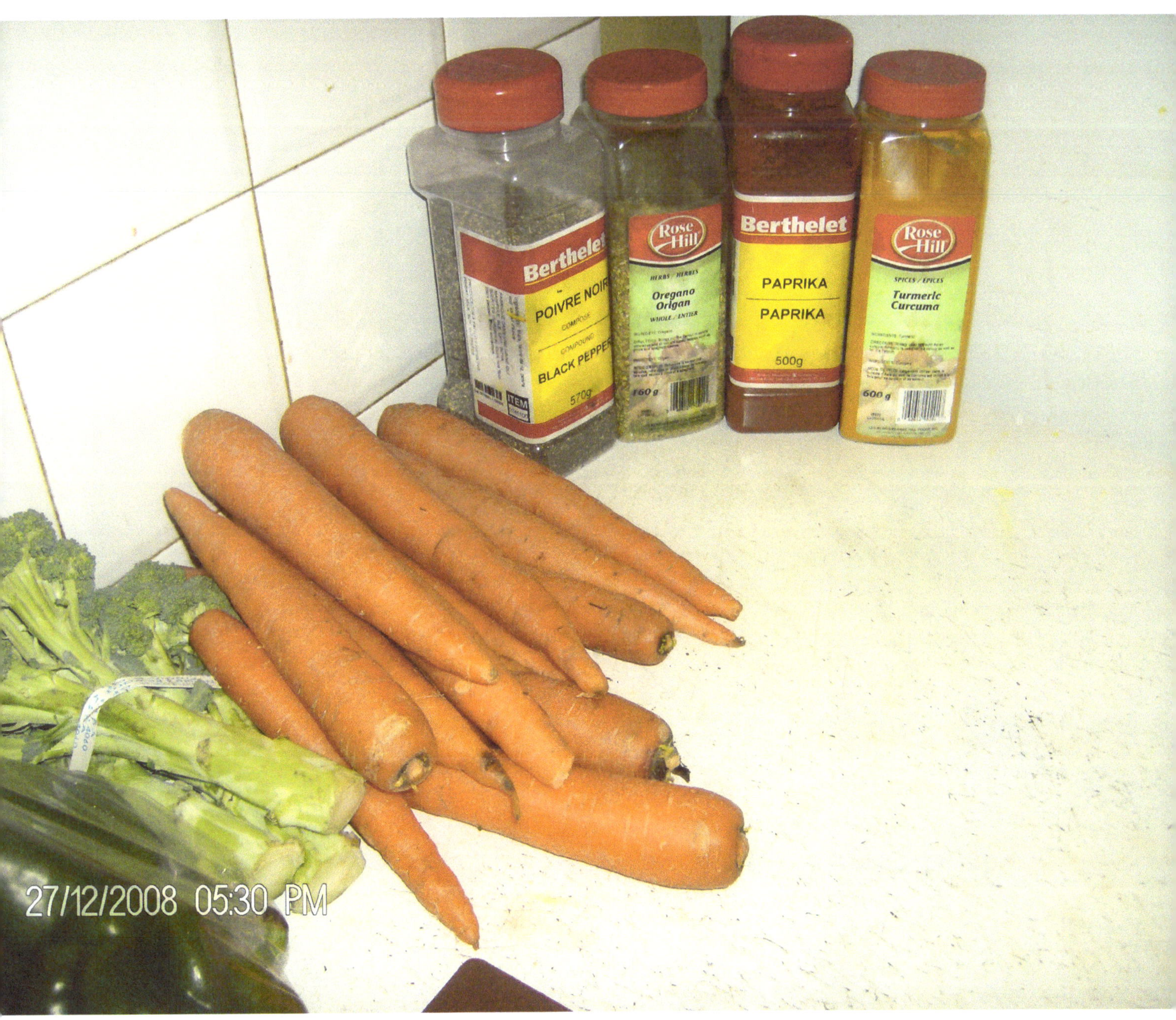
Berthelet
POIVRE NOIR
COMPOUND
BLACK PEPPE
570g
Rose Hill
HERBS / HERBES
Oregano
Origan
WHOLE / ENTIER
160 g
Berthelet
PAPRIKA
PAPRIKA
500g
Rose Hill
SPICES / EPICES
Turmeric
Curcuma
600 g
27/12/2008 05:30 PM

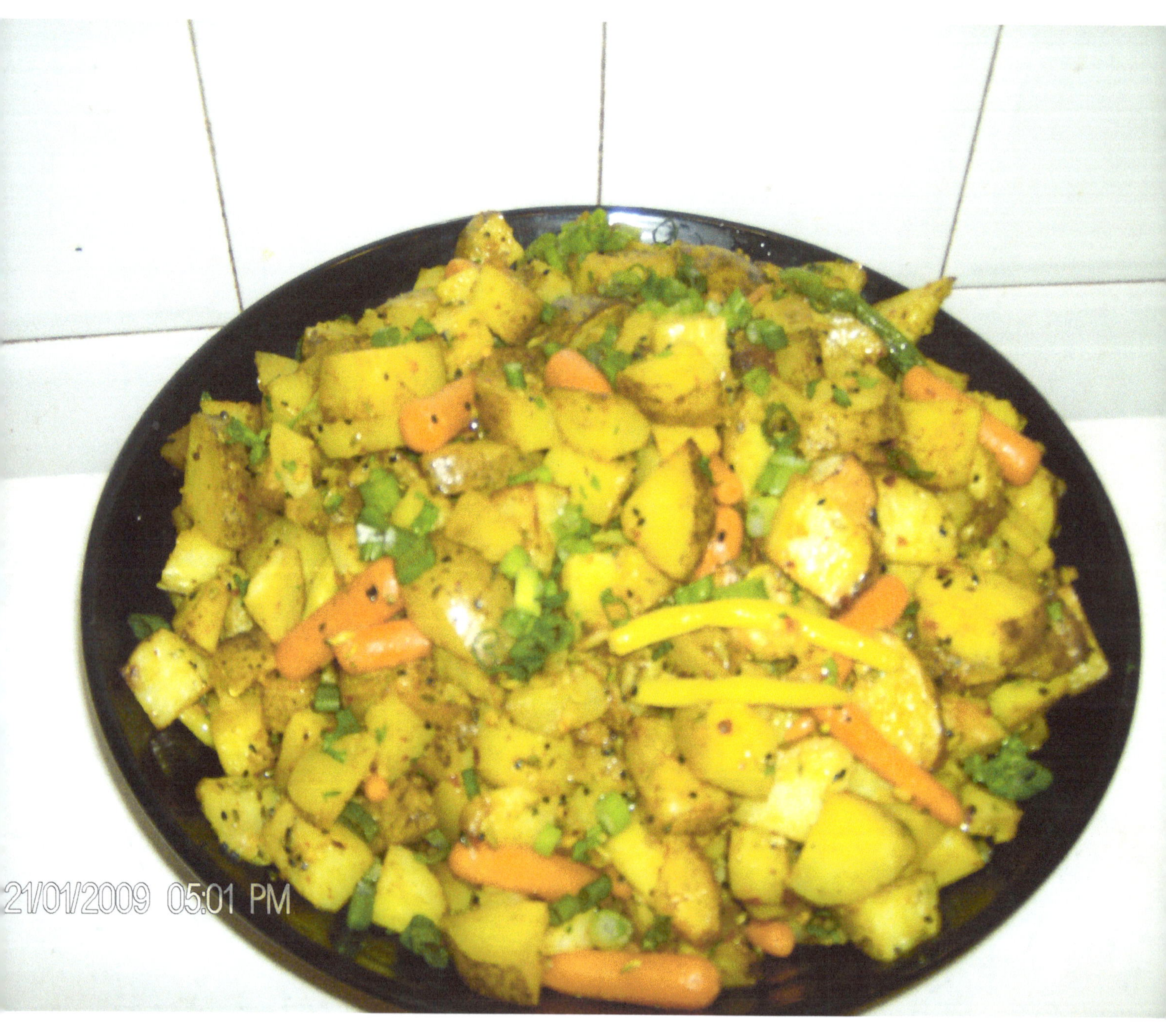
21/01/2009 05:01 PM

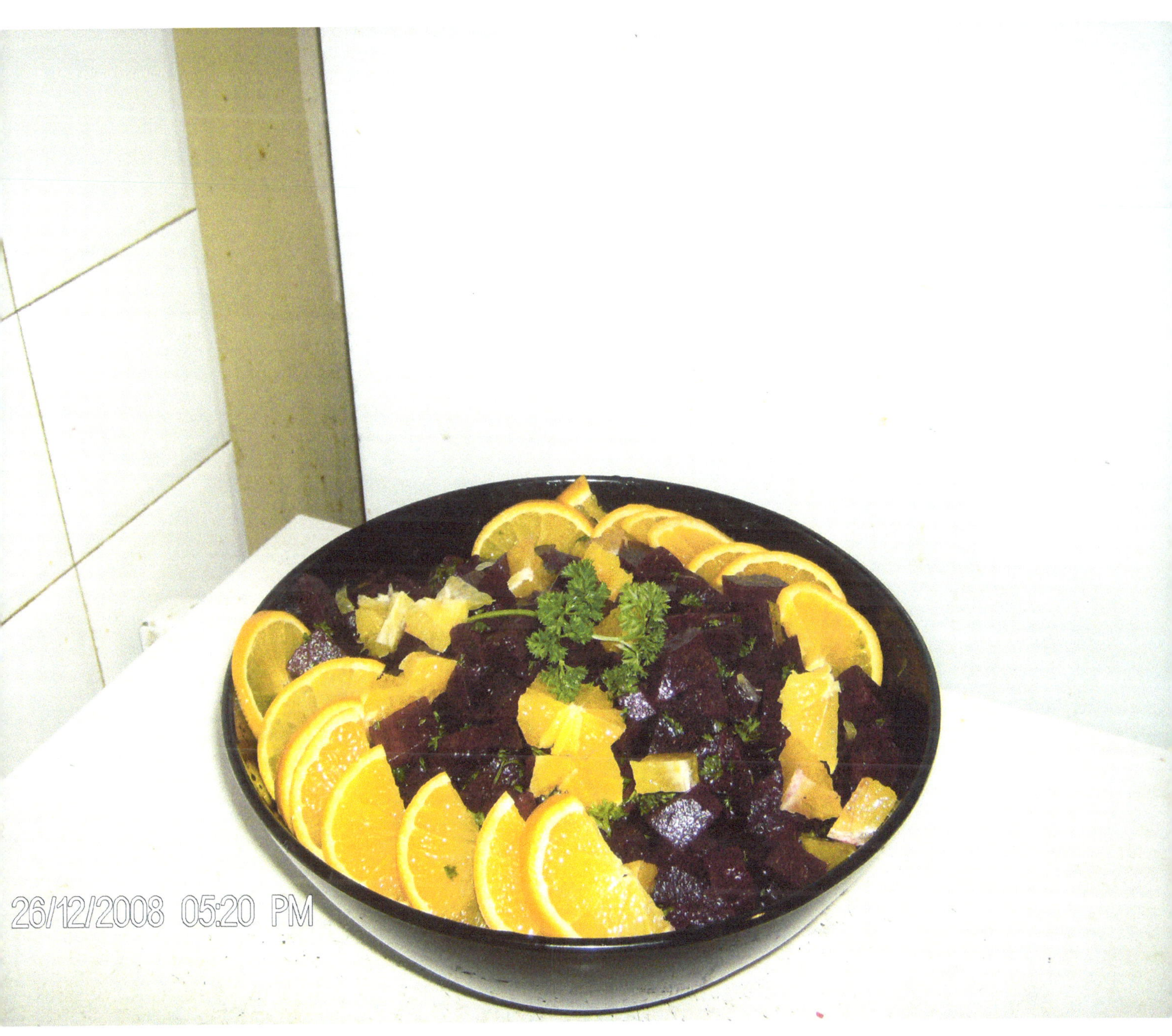
26/12/2008 05:20 PM

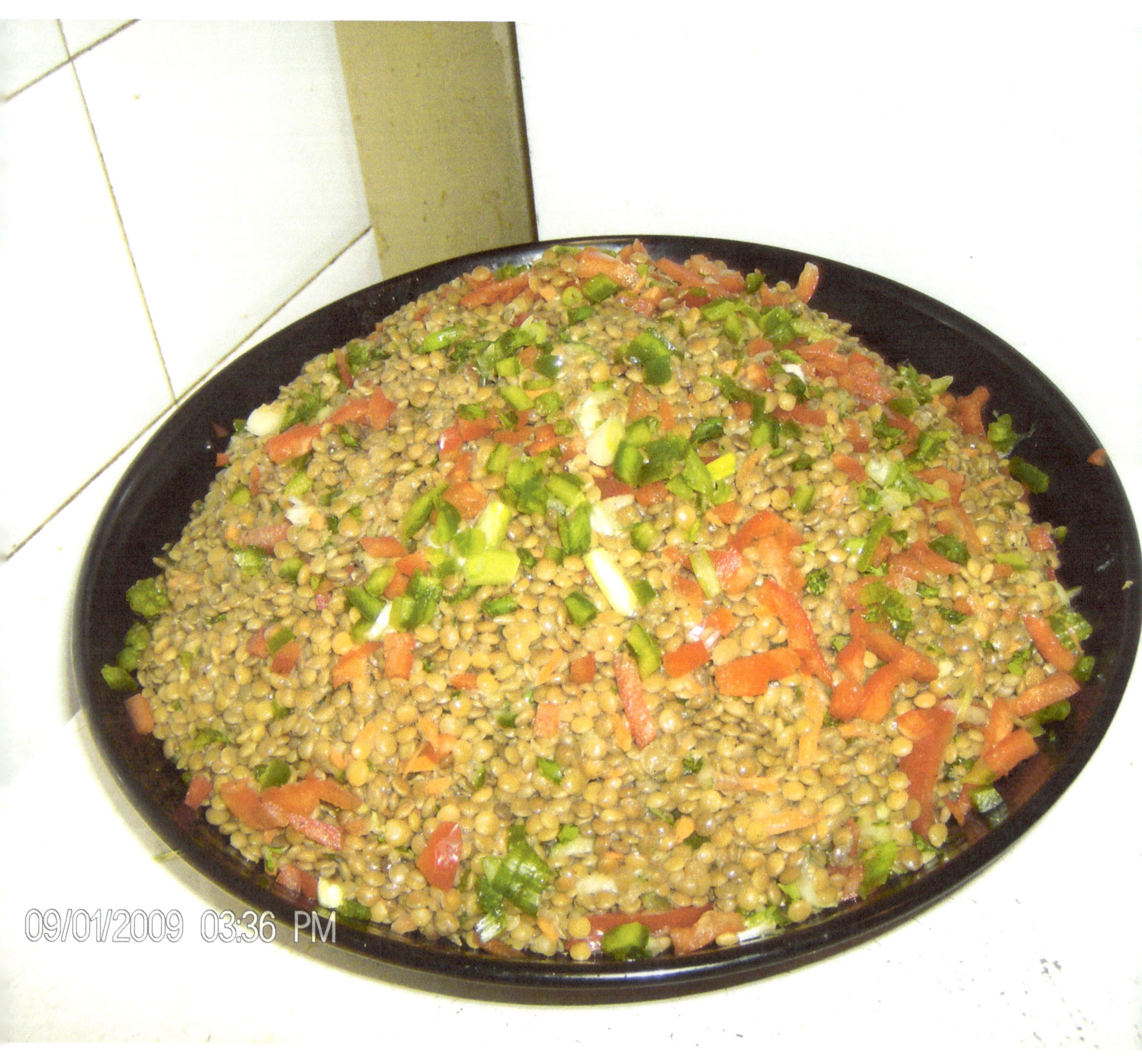
09/01/2009 03:36 PM

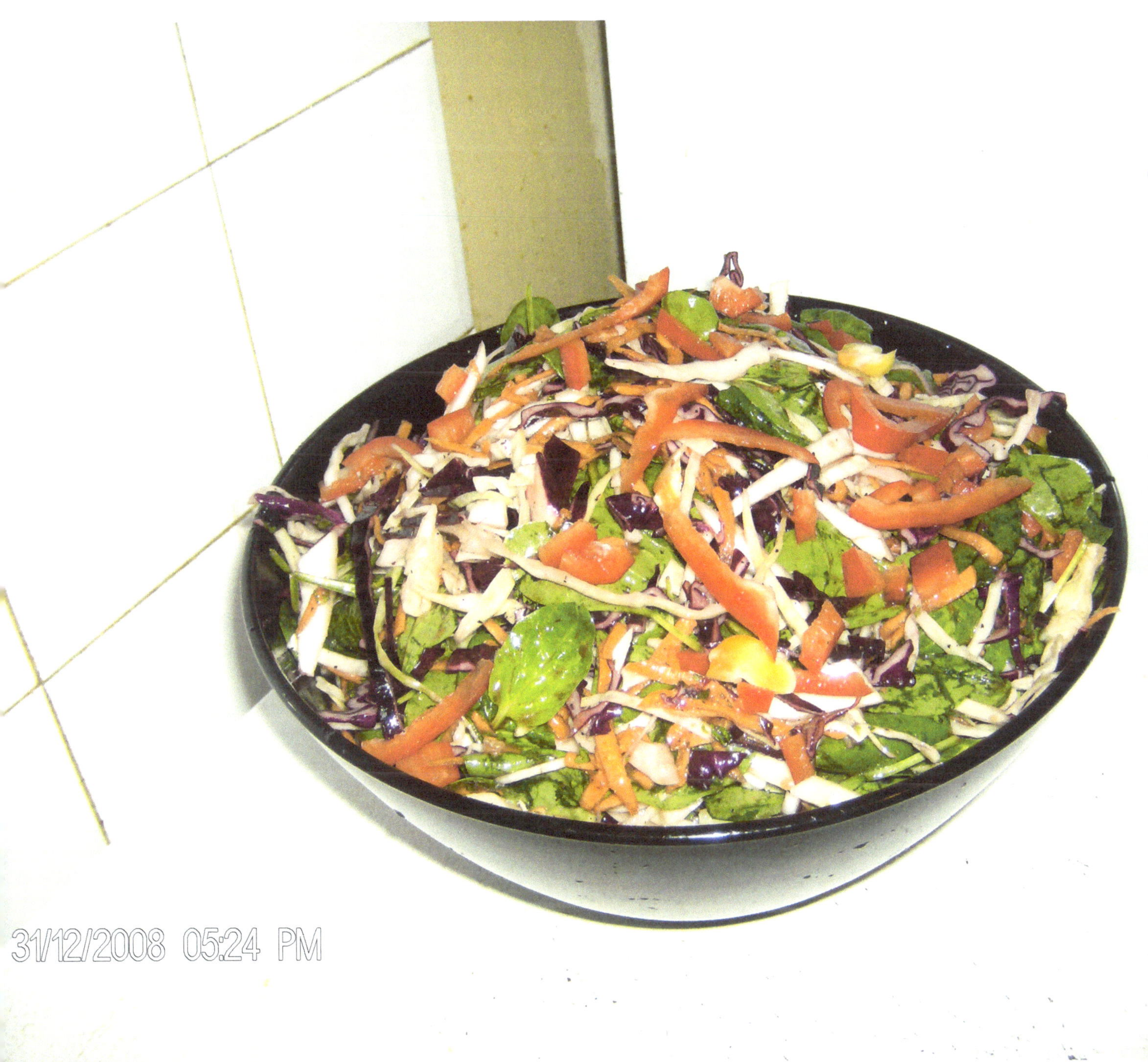
31/12/2008 05:24 PM

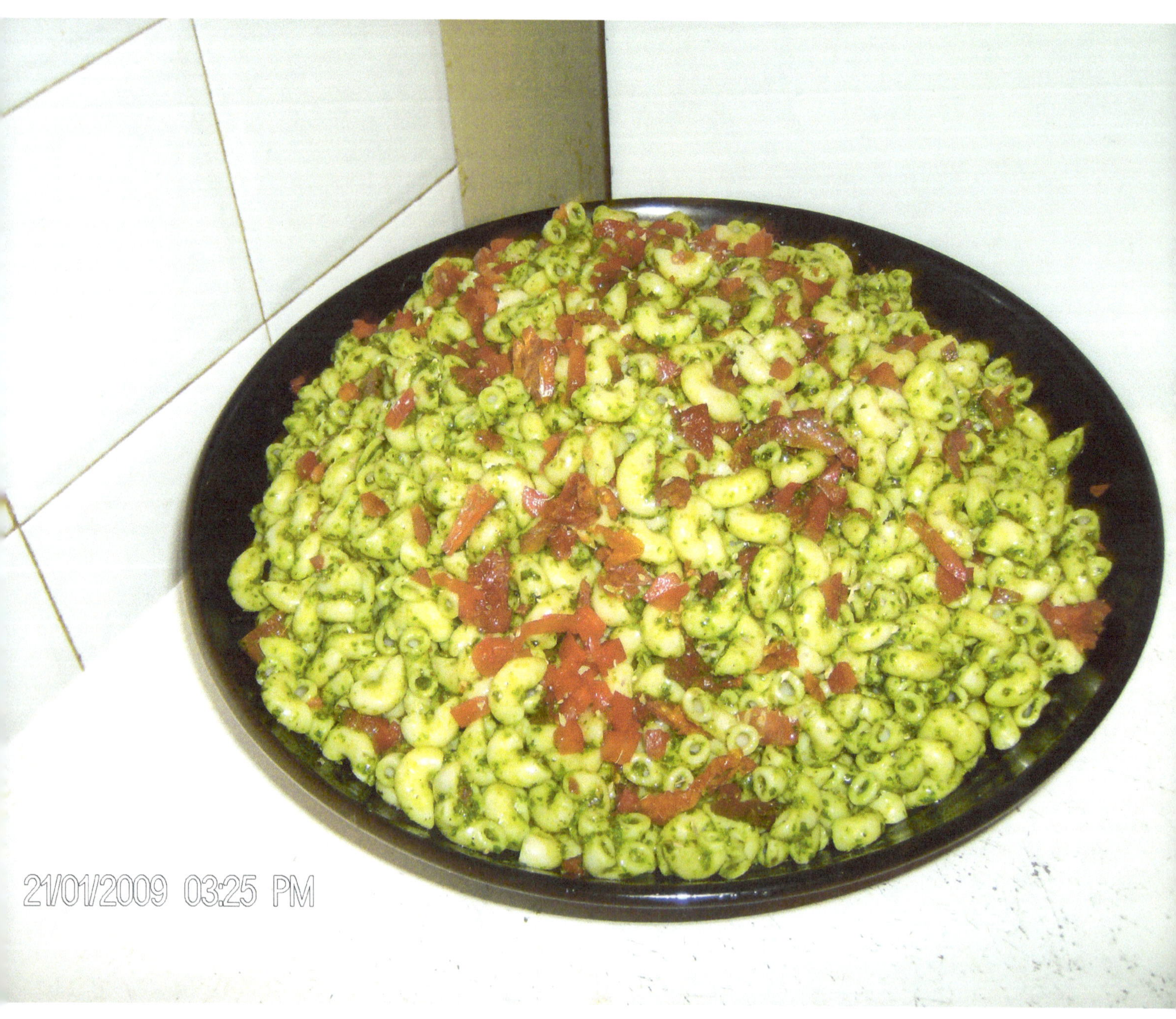
21/01/2009 03:25 PM

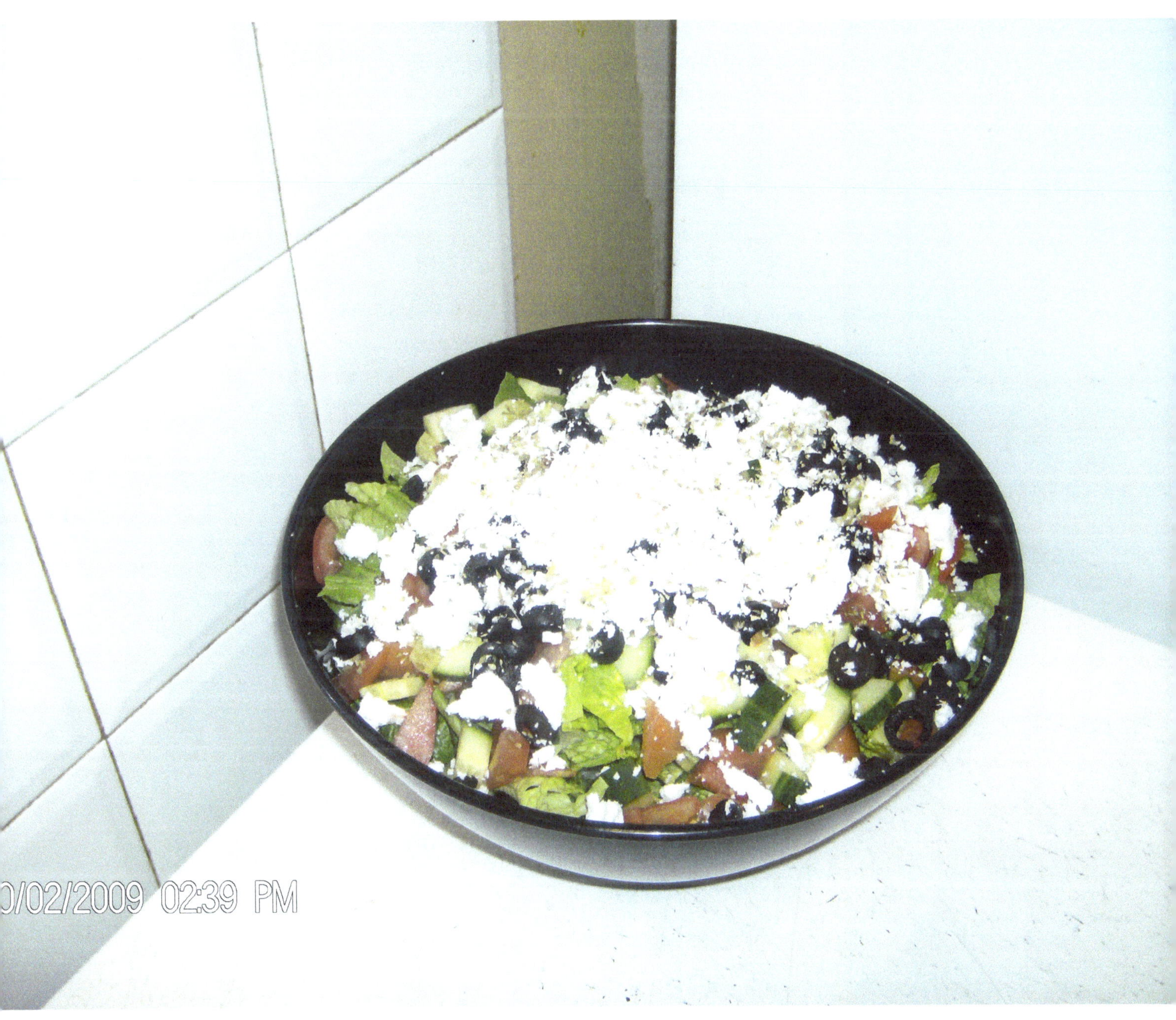
/02/2009 02:39 PM

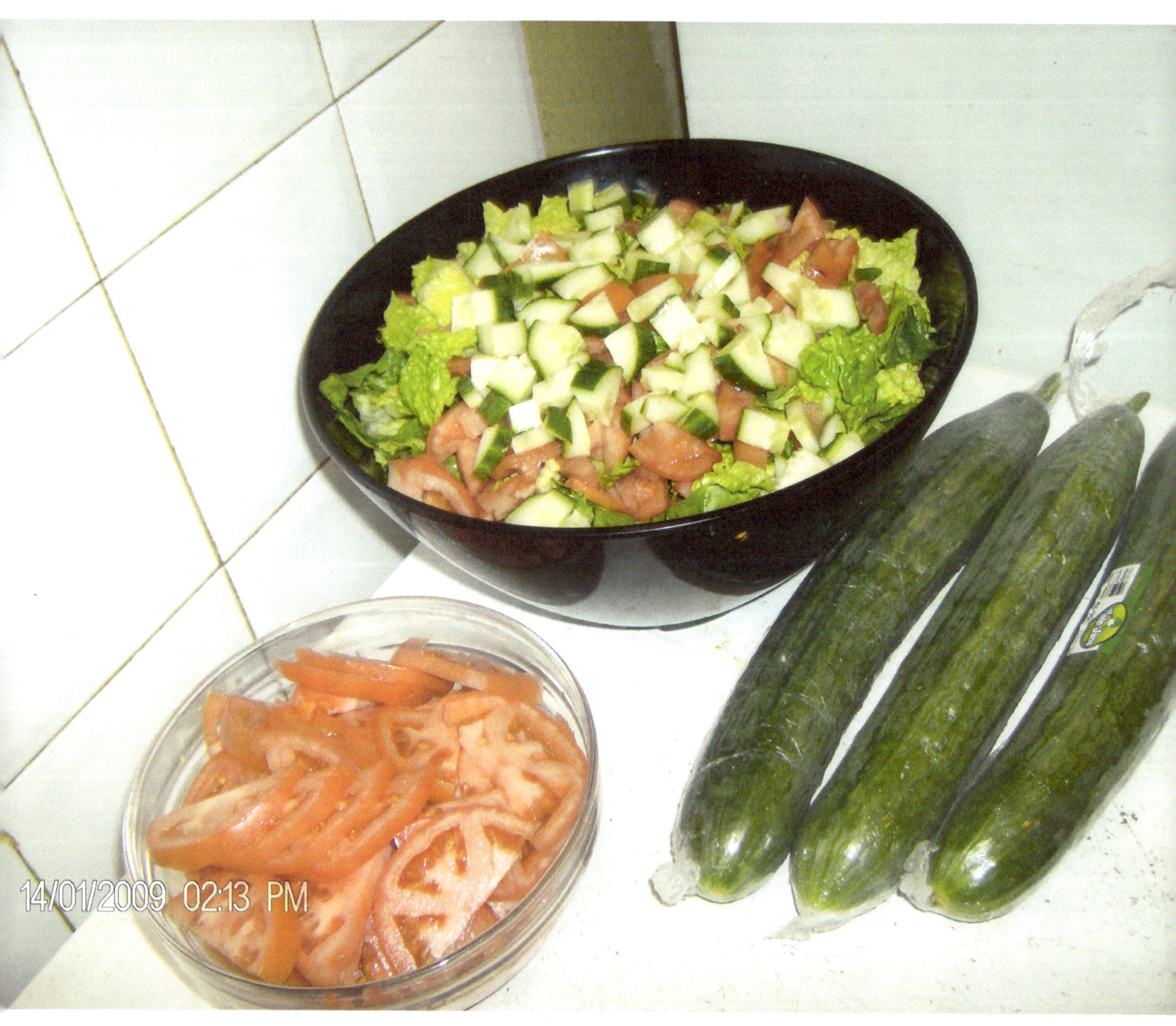
14/01/2009 02:13 PM

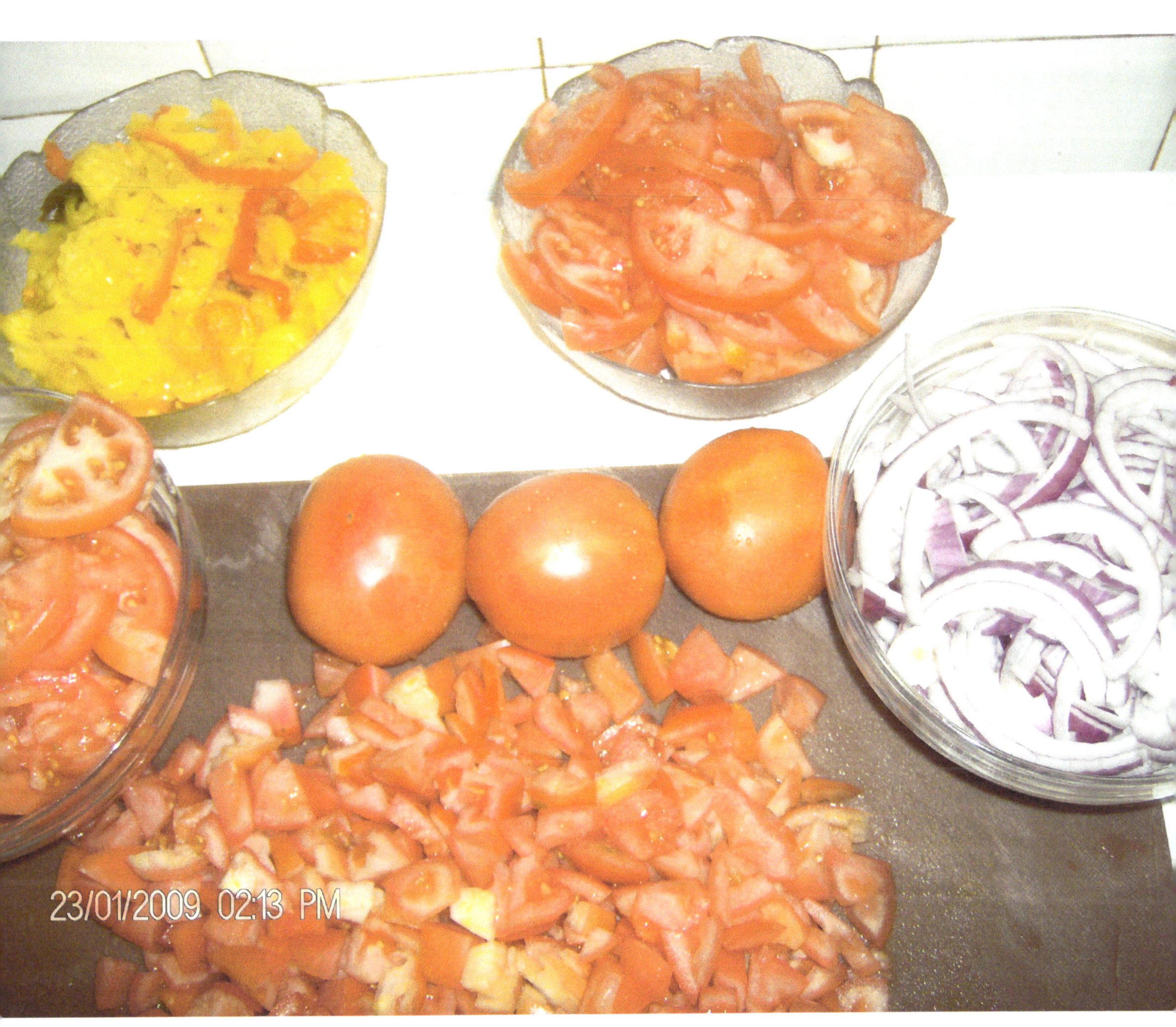
23/01/2009 02:13 PM

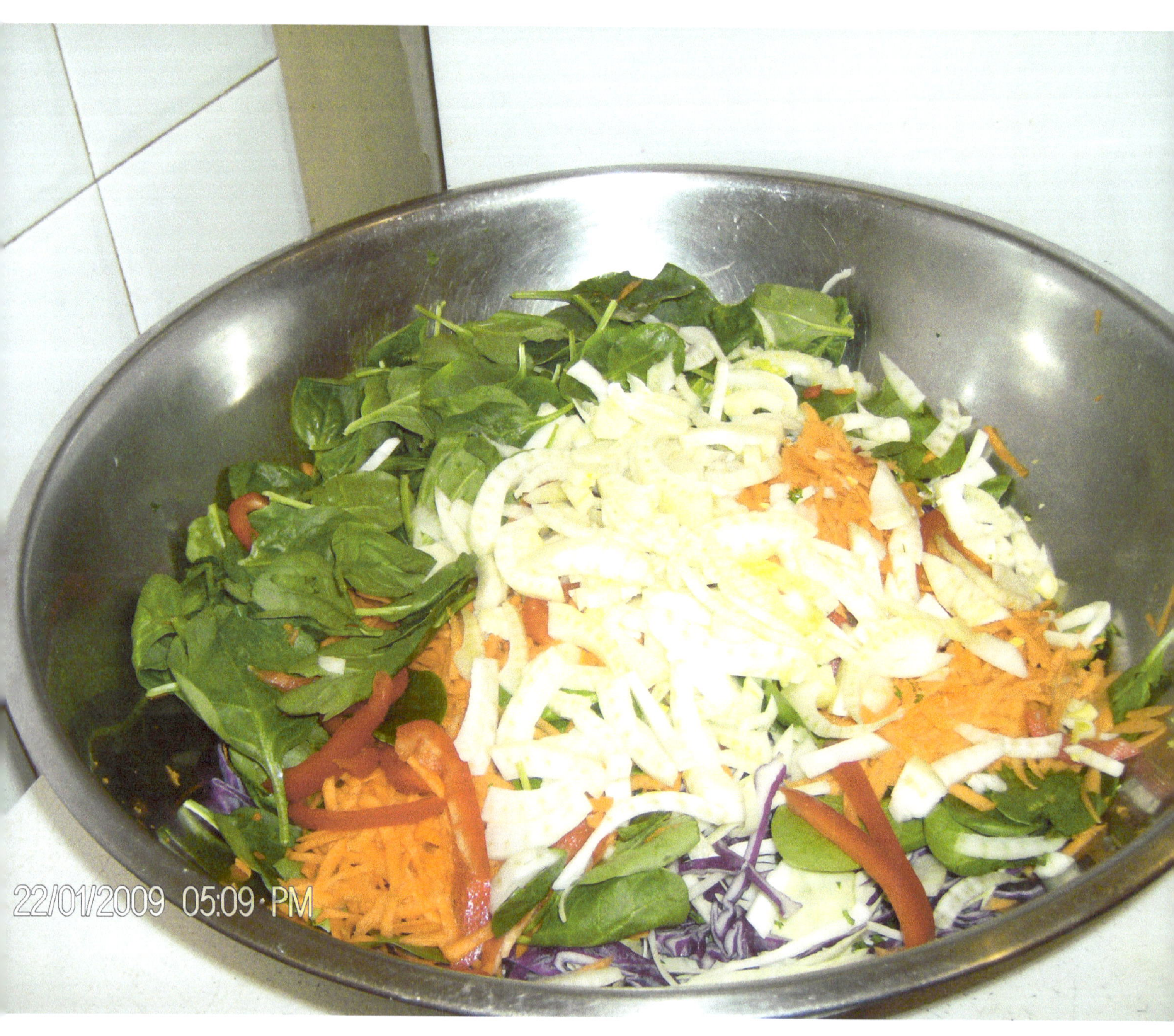
22/01/2009 05:09 PM

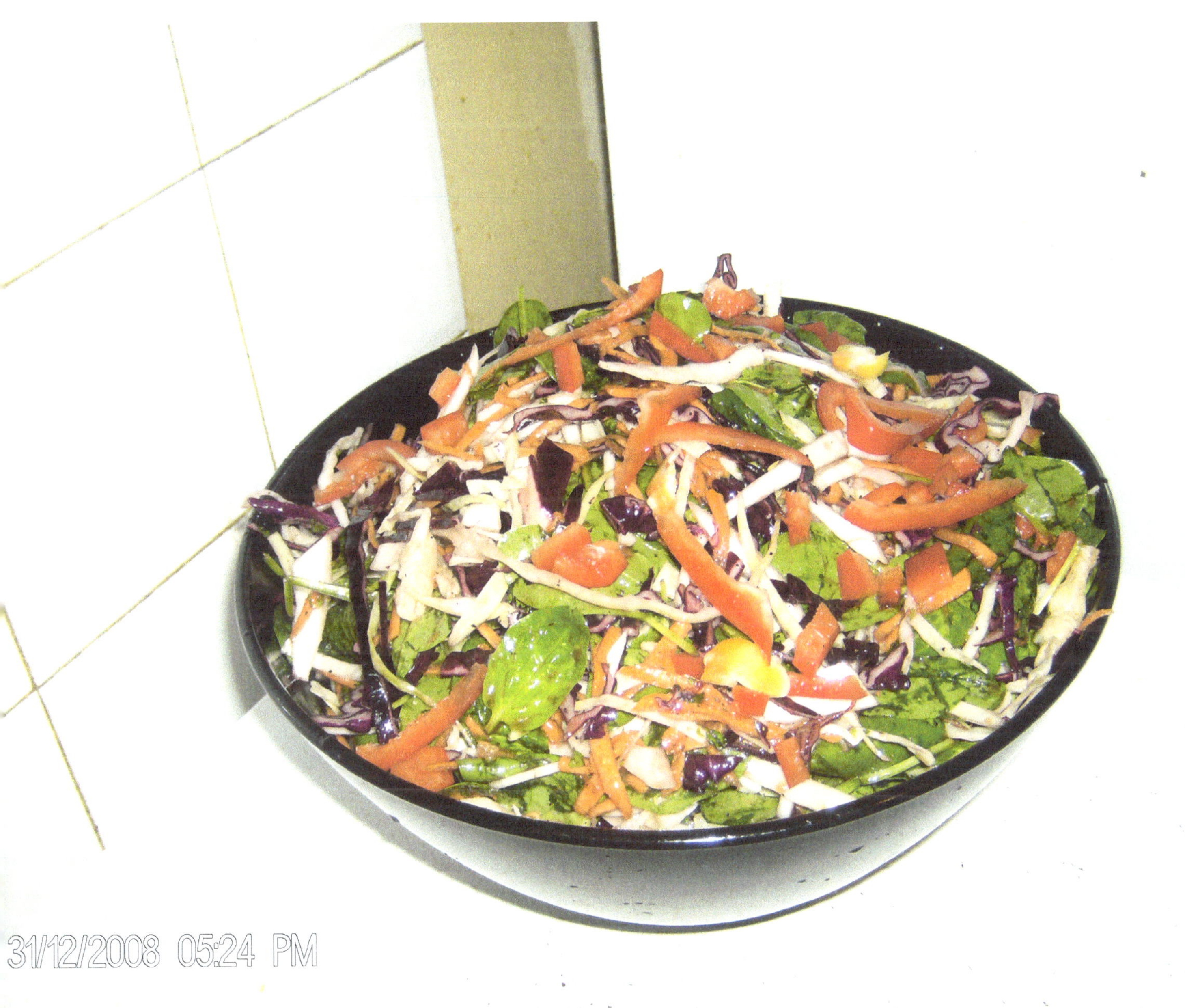
31/12/2008 05:24 PM

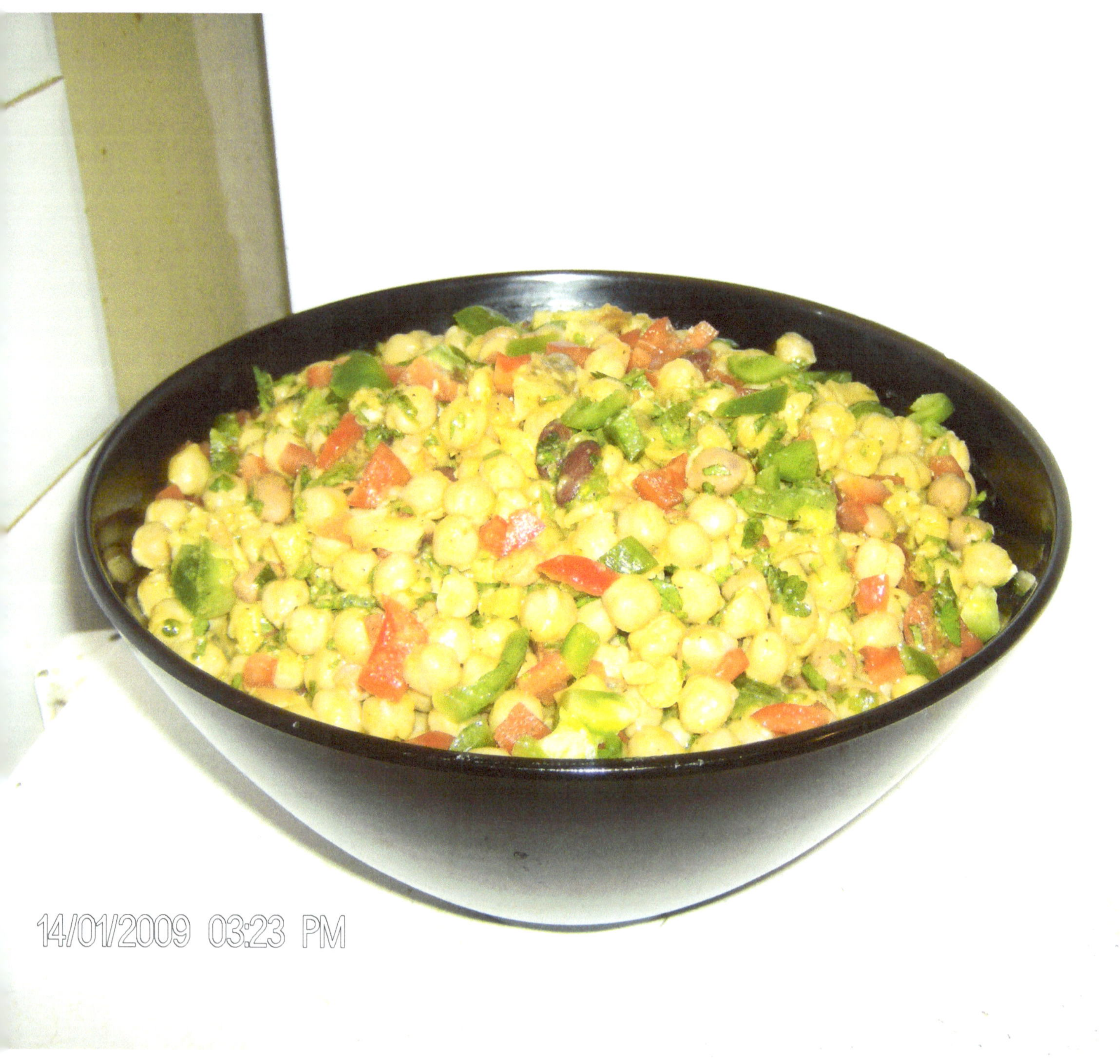
14/01/2009 03:23 PM

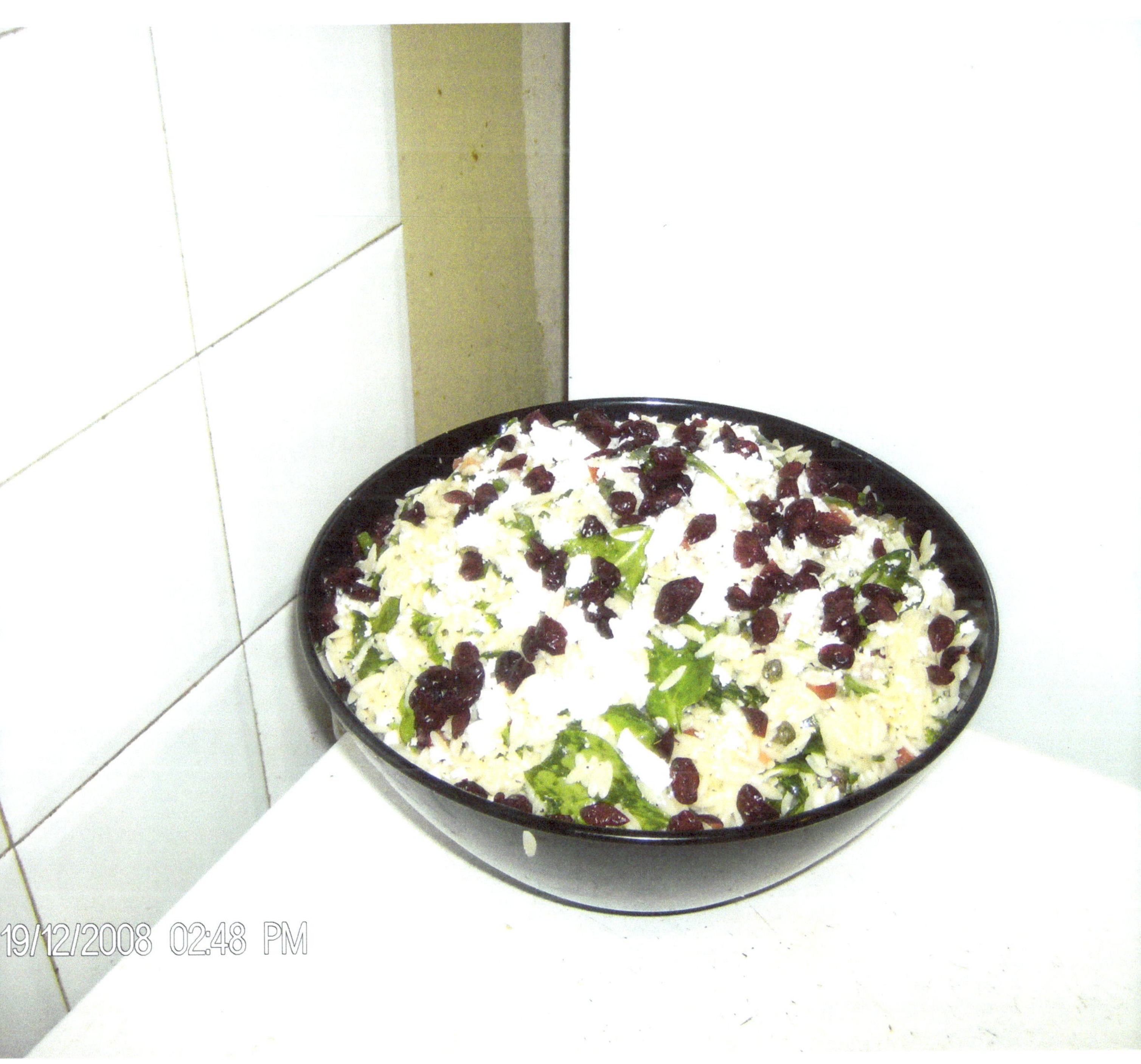
19/12/2008 02:48 PM

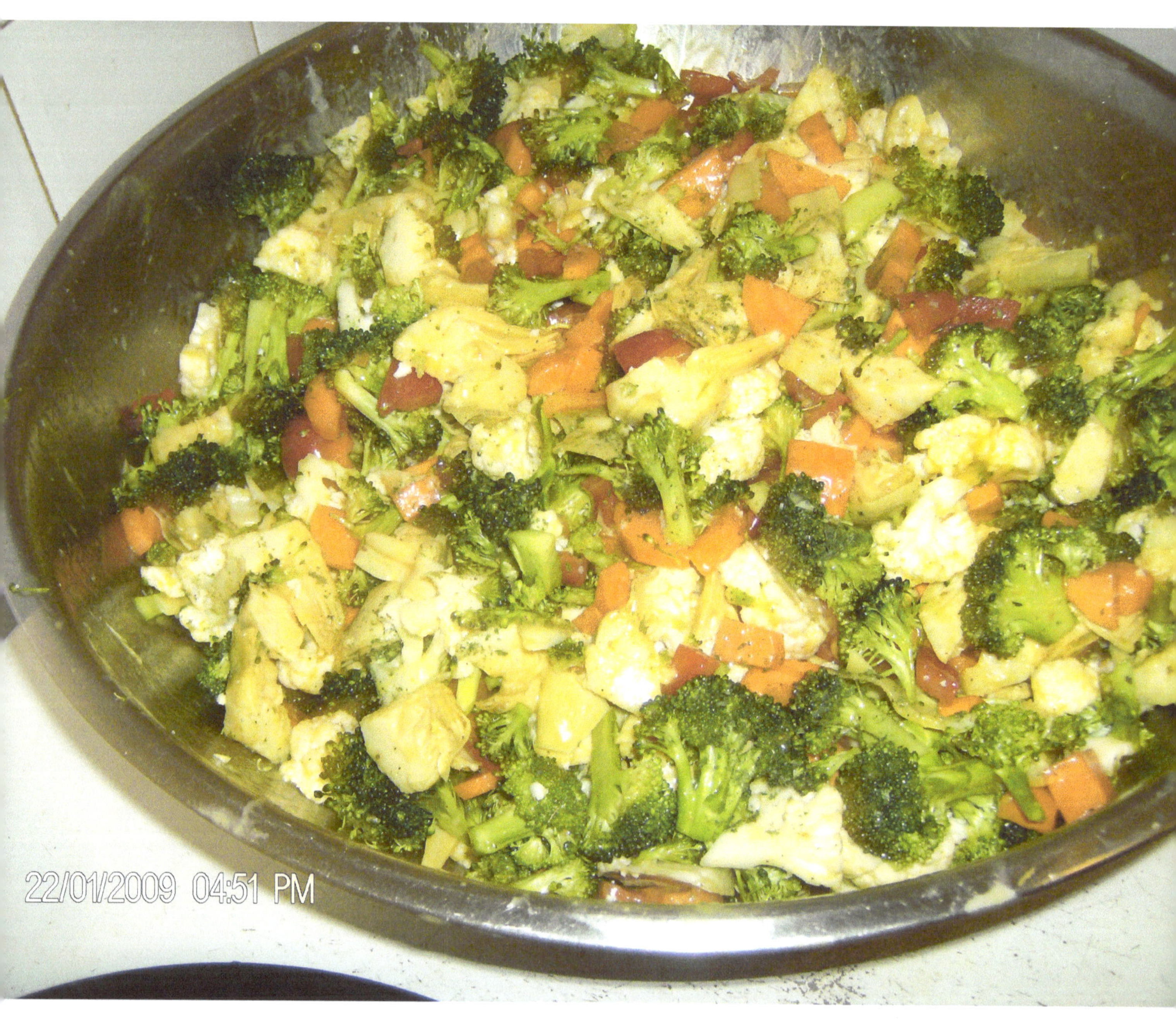
22/01/2009 04:51 PM

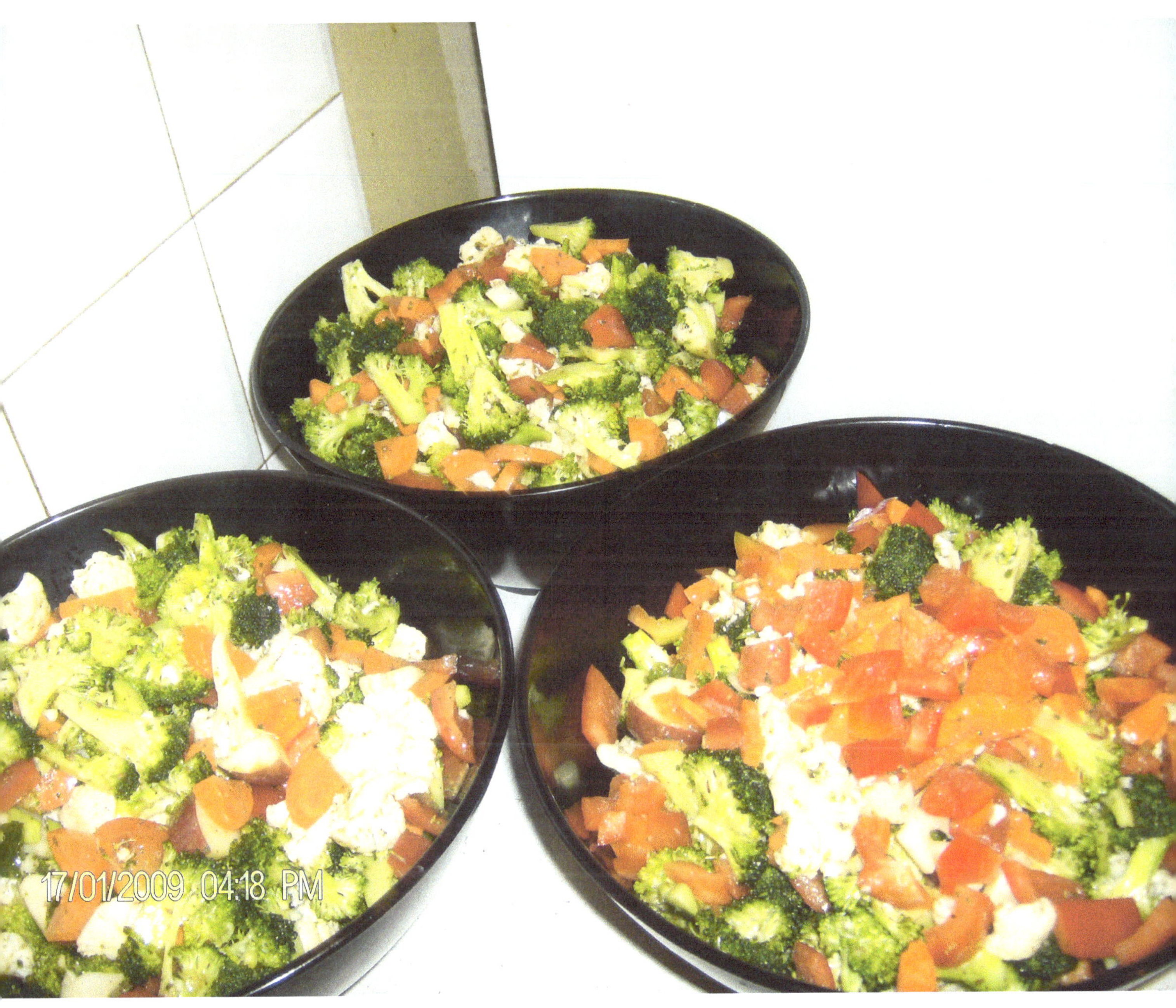
17/01/2009 04:18 PM

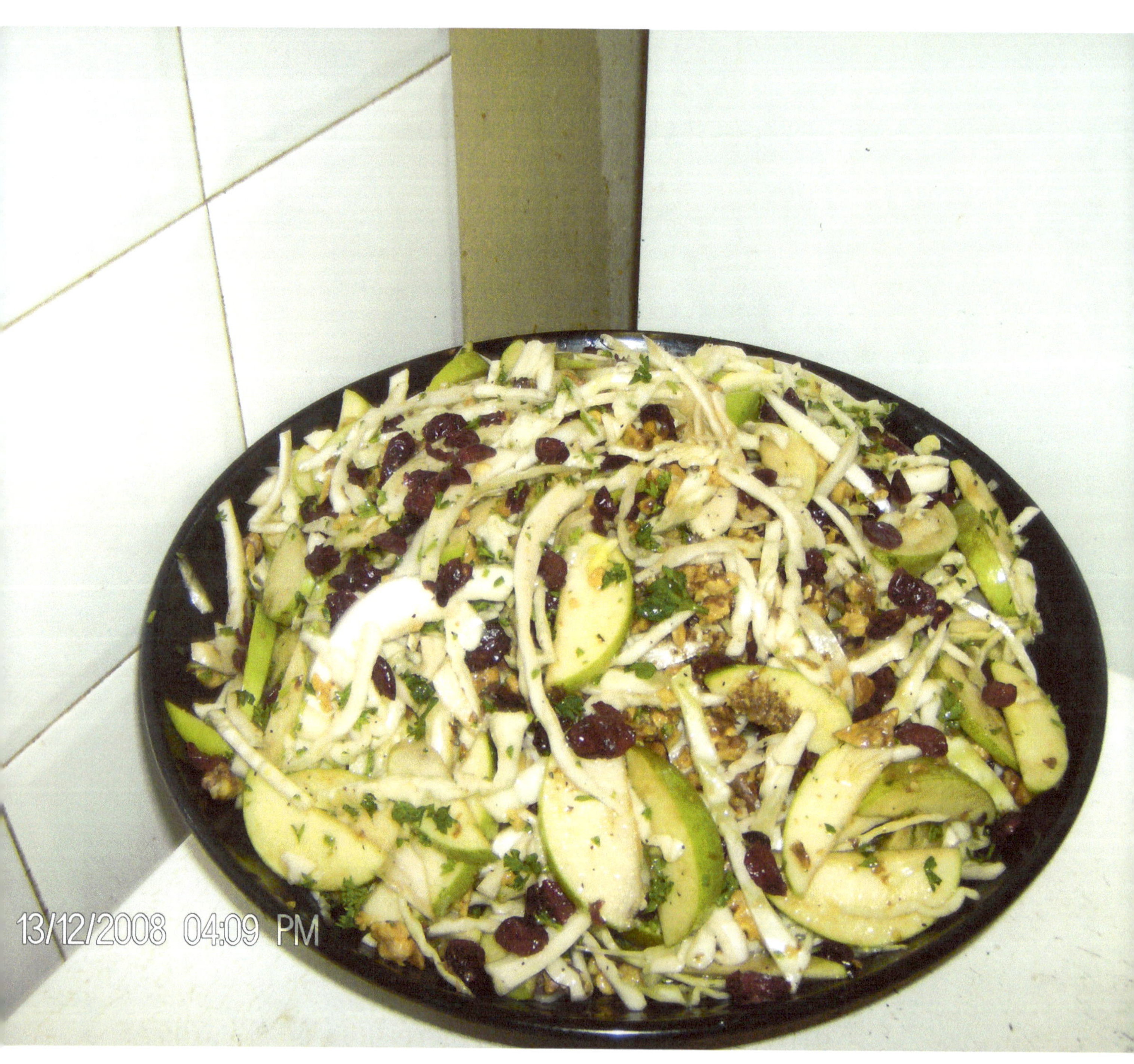
13/12/2008 04:09 PM

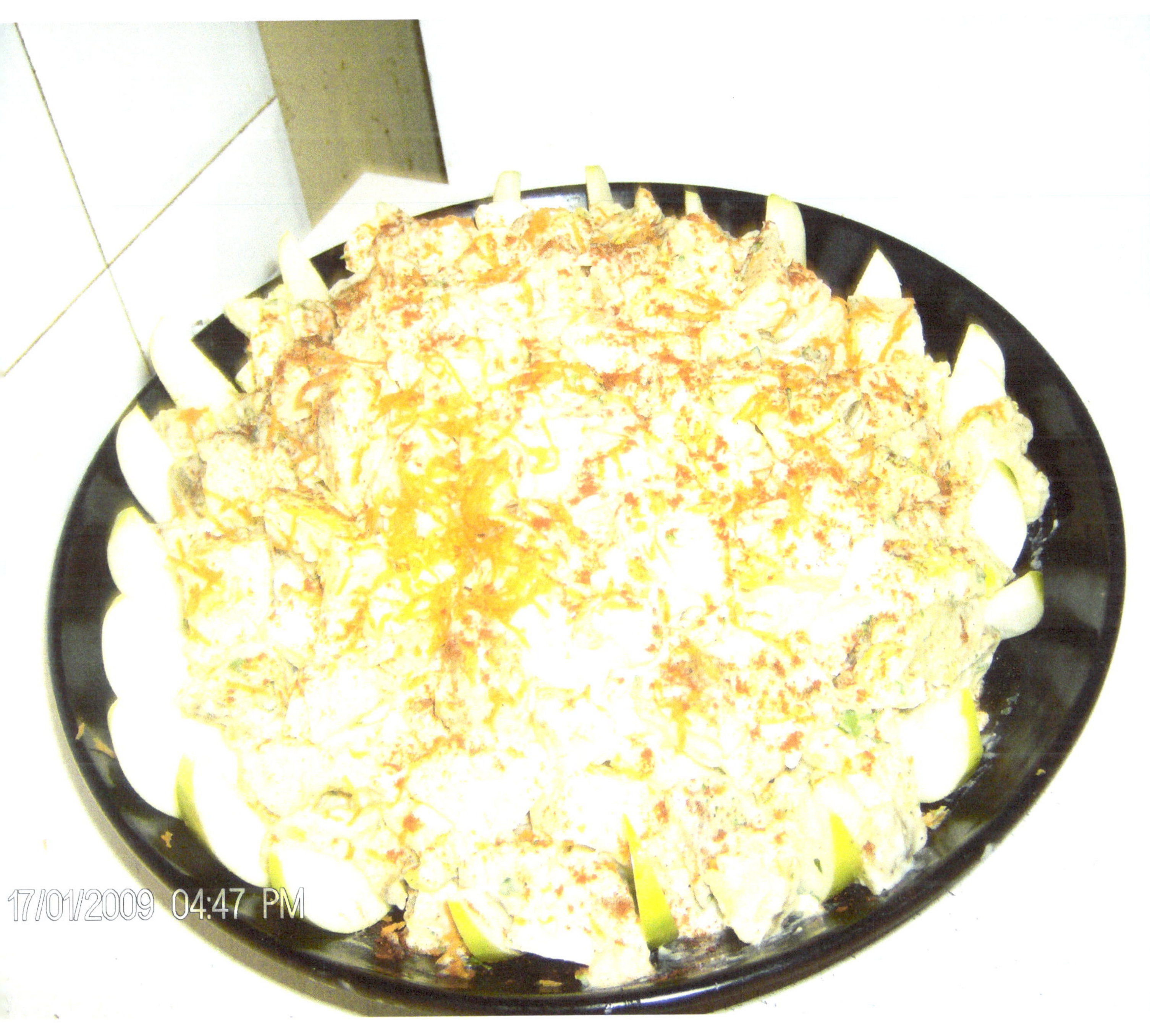
17/01/2009 04:47 PM

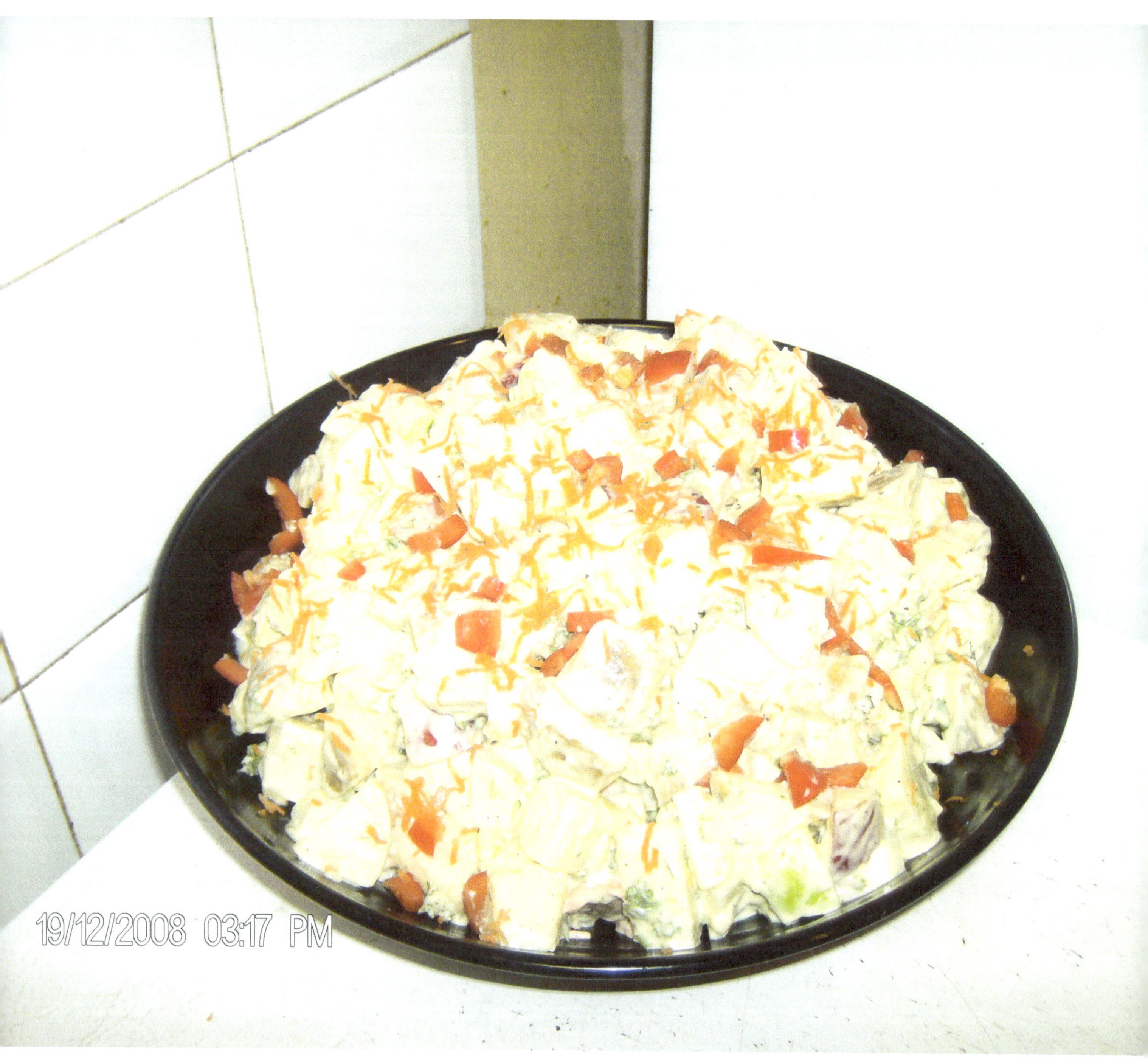
19/12/2008 03:17 PM

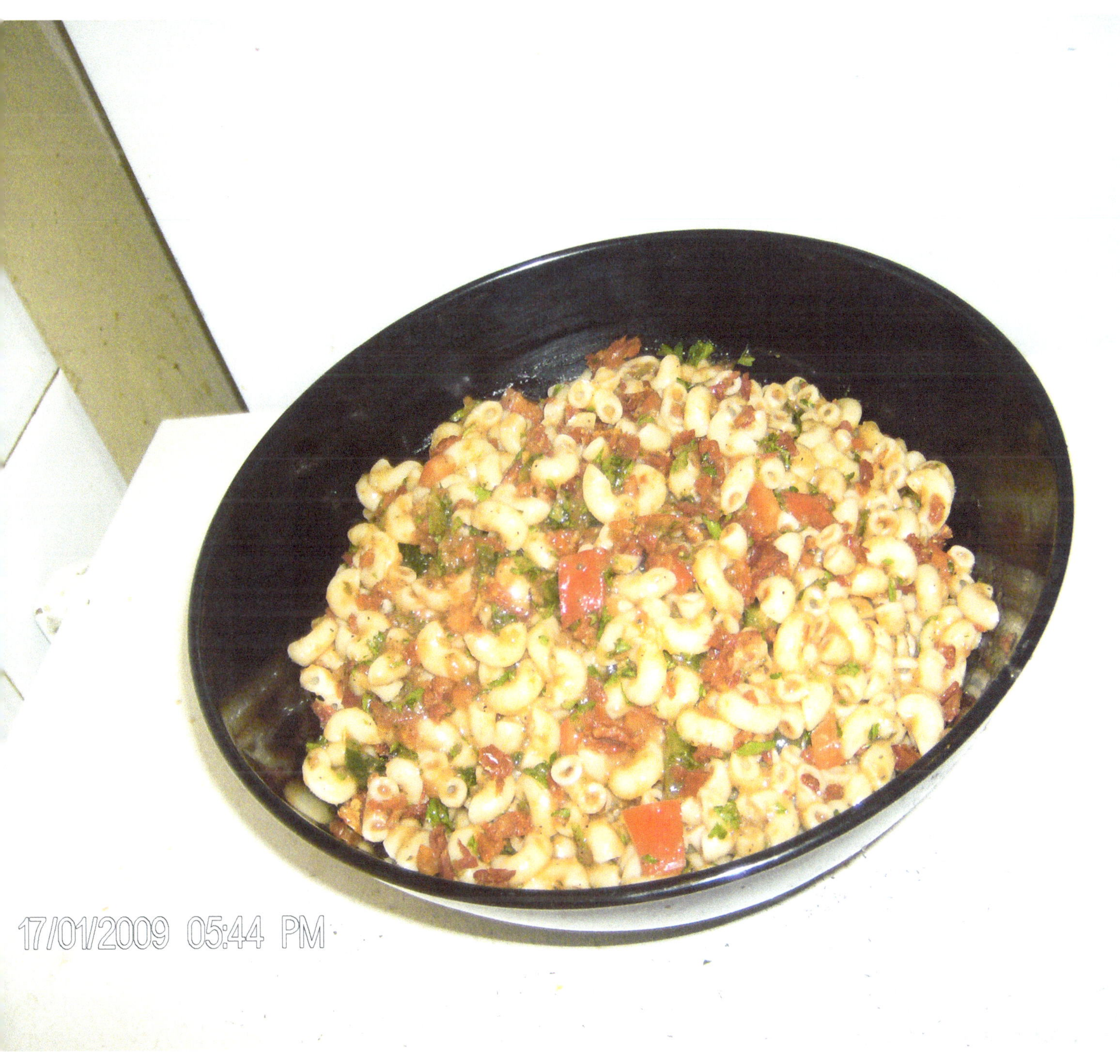
17/01/2009 05:44 PM

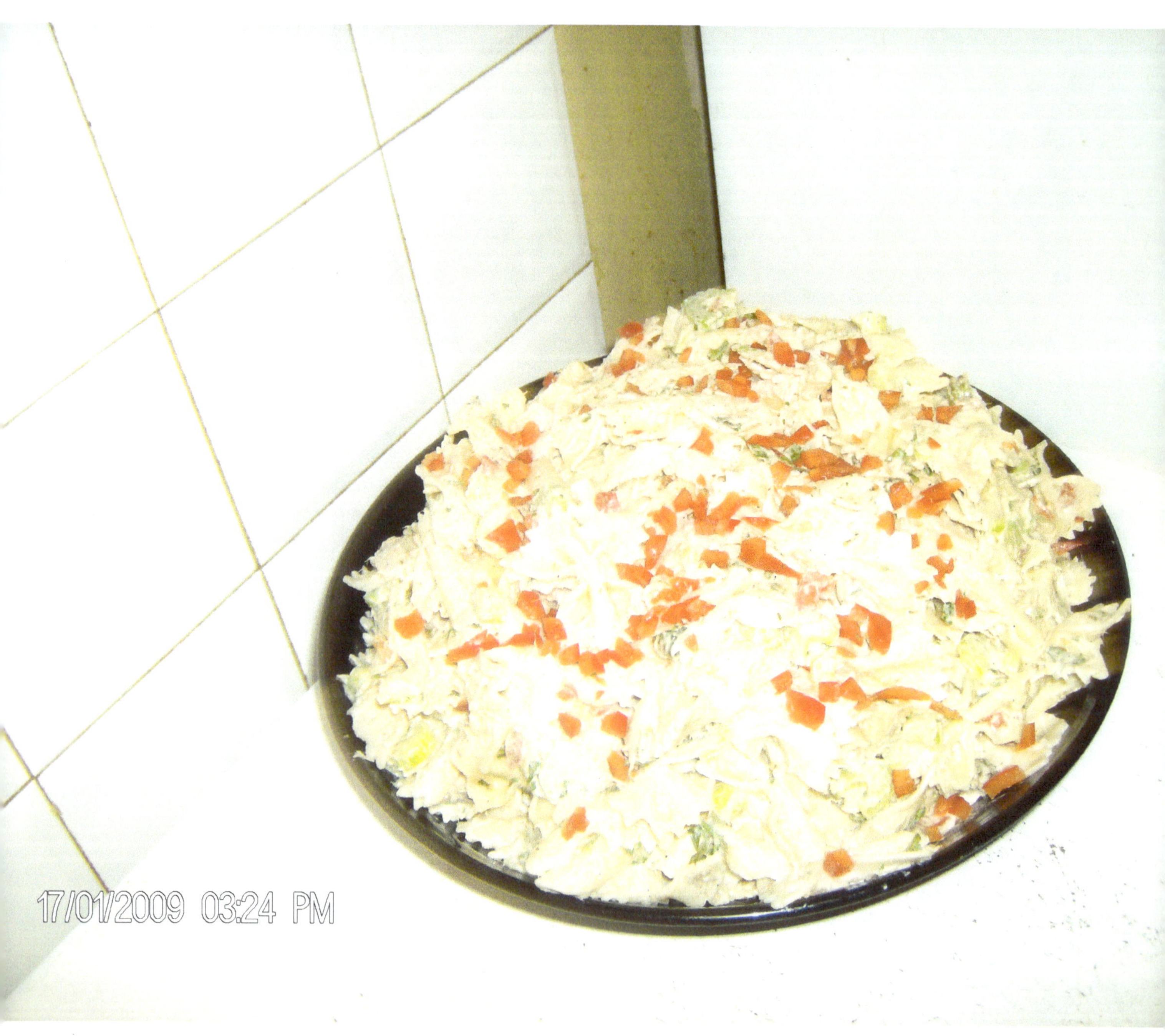
17/01/2009 03:24 PM

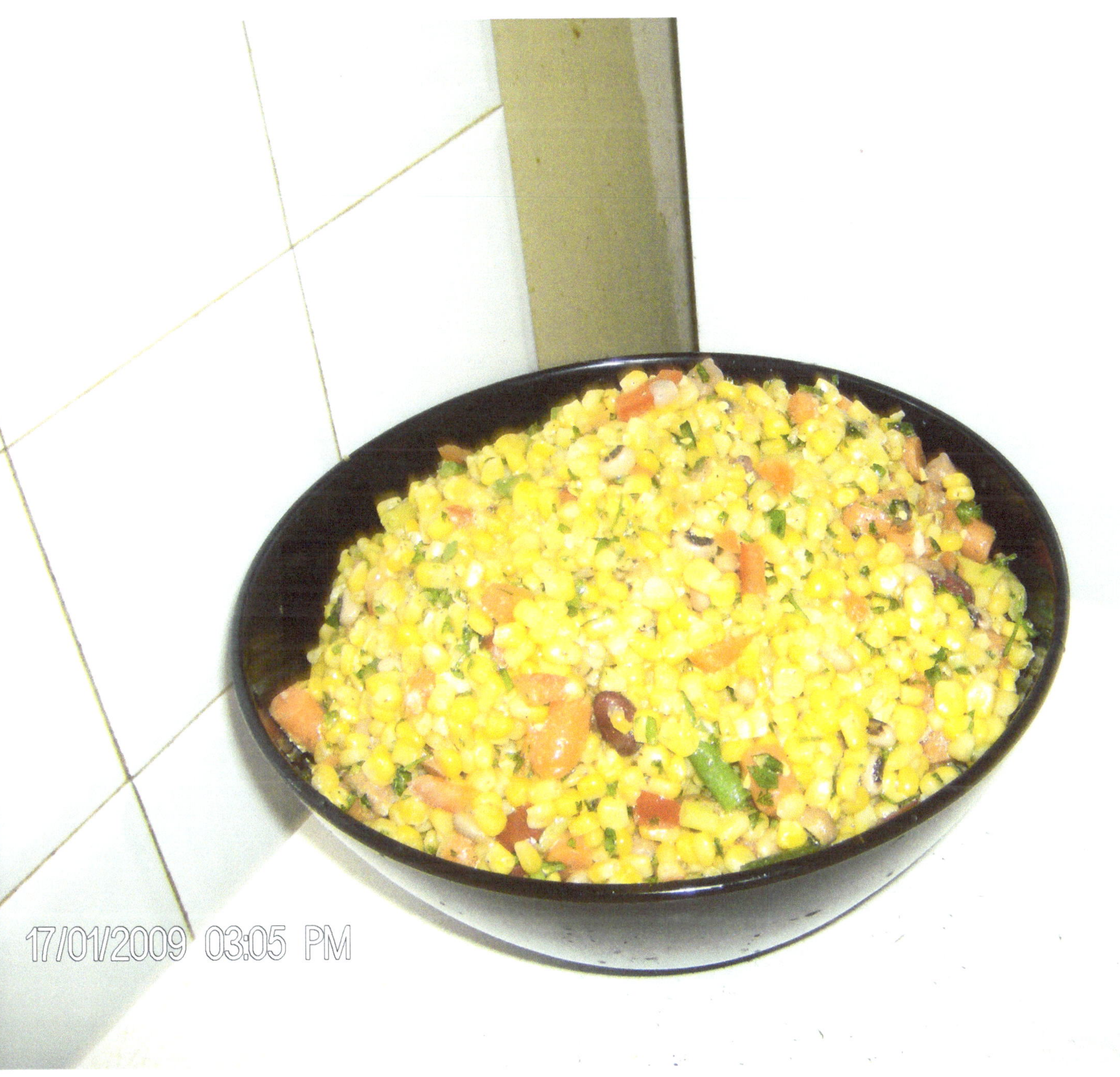
17/01/2009 03:05 PM

www.ingramcontent.com/pod-product-compliance
Lightning Source LLC
LaVergne TN
LVHW070150110826
845147LV00002B/365

* 9 7 8 1 4 2 6 9 3 5 5 5 8 *